THE MELATONIN MIRACLE

Nature's Age-Reversing, Disease-Fighting, Sex-Enhancing Hormone

Walter Pierpaoli, M.D., Ph.D.,
and William Regelson, M.D.,
with Carol Colman

POCKET BOOKS
New York   London   Toronto   Sydney   Tokyo   Singapore

POCKET BOOKS, a division of Simon & Schuster Inc.
1230 Avenue of the Americas, New York, NY 10020

ISBN: 978-1-4516-1312-4

First Pocket Books printing April 1996

10 9 8 7 6 5 4 3

POCKET and colophon are registered trademarks of Simon & Schuster Inc.

Printed in the U.S.A.

To my parents Giuseppina and Mario Pierpaoli to whom I owe the genetics of my body, mind, and soul, and also my endurance and the capacity to suffer and to love. I am also deeply indebted to the skeptics whose challenges are now answered in the evidence of the aging clock.

—WP

To Anna Regelson and Sylvia Phillips Regelson.

—WR

The ideas, procedures, and suggestions contained in this book are not intended to replace the services of a trained health professional. All matters regarding your health require medical supervision. If you have any preexisting medical conditions, you should consult your physician before adopting the suggestions and procedures in this book. Any applications of the treatments set forth in this book are at the reader's discretion. If you are taking prescription medication on a regular basis, please check with your physician before using melatonin. In some cases, melatonin may enhance the effect of certain types of medication, so you may need to reduce your dosages accordingly.

Appendix 1, from *Proc. Natl. Acad. Sci. USA* 91:787–791, is reprinted by permission of The National Academy of Science.
Appendix 2, from Pierpaoli, *The Aging Clock*, is reprinted by permission of The New York Academy of Sciences.

ACKNOWLEDGMENTS

This book would be unthinkable without the outstanding skill, enthusiasm, and very hard work of the writer Carol Colman and the personal involvement and brilliant vision of our editor, Laurie Bernstein. Grateful acknowledgment to our agent, Barbara Lowenstein. Special thanks also to Owen Davies for his contribution and start-up efforts. We owe much of the inspiration of Walter's work on aging to his beloved friend, the late Vladimir Dilman of St. Petersburg, Russia, whose concept on the decay of central hypothalamic feedback regulation during aging anticipated by decades the aging clock. We also wish to thank Ashley Montagu, whose intuition was pivotal and very much appreciated. In addition we would like to mention Nicola Fabris, Gonzague Kistler, Novera Spector, Changxian Yi, Vladimir Lesnikov, E. Mocchegiani, Samuel McCann, and all the dear colleagues at INRCA, Ancona, for our common aim to defeat aging in order to live better.

Walter acknowledges Annemarie, Ezra, and Sarah Pierpaoli, and Gualberto Gualerni, who have shared and continue to share the complex vicissitudes of his life. He is grateful to God for his wife Lisa, who was with him during the very dark days in Ticino, Switzerland, where the evidence for the aging clock first emerged.

Bill acknowledges the help of Don Yarborough and Sen. Alan Cranston, whose efforts made possible the FIBER that drew many scientists together to stimulate research in the biology of aging.

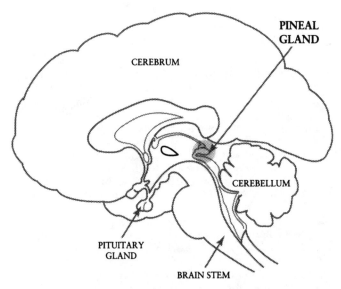

PINEAL
GLAND

CEREBRUM

CEREBELLUM

PITUITARY
GLAND

BRAIN STEM

*Diagram of the brain, highlighting the pineal gland
which produces melatonin.*

CONTENTS

Contents

Contents

PART THREE
Nature's Sex-Enhancing Hormone and Other Benefits of Melatonin   179

A NOTE TO READERS

In this book, we will tell you how melatonin can help you to "grow" young (Part One), remain disease free (Part Two), retain your sexual vitality, get a better night's sleep, and enhance the quality of your life in a variety of other ways (Part Three). We know that as you learn more about how melatonin actually performs these "miracles" you will be eager to know precisely how you can take melatonin in order to achieve each of these benefits. We want you to know that all of the necessary information on dosages along with precise instructions on when and how to take it are provided for you in Chapter 14.

FOREWORD

On June 4, 1993, a group of fifty distinguished scientists from all over the world gathered on Stromboli, an idyllic island off the coast of Italy, to participate in the Third Annual Stromboli Conference on Aging and Cancer.* The men and women who joined us that day say they found the air unforgettably charged, a condition that some might attribute to the effect of the island's ancient volcano, which still erupts (gently) at fifteen-minute intervals, the way it has for many thousands of years. We, however, prefer to think that although the ageless volcano was the appropriate backdrop for the conference, the true source of the electricity in the air was the startling scientific breakthrough that brought these preeminent scholars, physicians, and medical researchers together.

This discovery holds the very real promise that within our lifetimes we will be able to delay, and even reverse, the aging process, and that we will be able to prolong life not by mere years, but by decades. Moreover, we will live those added decades in a body that is healthy, vigorous, and youthful.

* The papers that were presented at this conference are published in *The Aging Clock: The Pineal Gland and Other Pacemakers in the Progression of Aging and Carcinogenesis—Third Stromboli Conference on Aging and Cancer* (NATO Advanced Research Workshop No. 920909), Annals of the New York Academy of Sciences, Vol. 719, May 31, 1994 (Walter Pierpaoli, William Regelson, and Nicola Fabris, eds.).

For those of us who organized it, the five-day conference marked the culmination of decades of study and research, during which our view of the aging process was radically transformed. As we shared our findings with the conference participants, so was theirs. Now, before more time passes, we want to share our findings with you. We are convinced that after reading this book, your view of the aging process will also be radically transformed.

At the Stromboli conference, we presented our discovery of what we call the "aging clock," the center in the brain that controls the aging process. We also presented the results of our work with melatonin, the remarkable hormone that is produced by the aging clock and that functions as its chemical messenger. We explained that the aging clock, through its messenger, melatonin, tells our body when to age. We showed that melatonin, which can be purchased without a prescription in synthetic form in neighborhood pharmacies and natural food stores, can extend life and can help prevent many of the debilitating physical and mental illnesses that have become all too synonymous with aging. In this book, you will learn much more about the aging clock and what we have come to call the melatonin miracle.

Before we continue, however, I would like to tell you something about us, the authors of this book. First, I would like to introduce you to the man who convened the Stromboli Conference on Aging and Cancer, the man who is revolutionizing the way we view aging, my colleague and coauthor, Walter Pierpaoli, M.D., Ph.D. Walter is the director of the Biancalana-Masera Foundation for the Aged in Ancona, Italy, one of the most innovative research centers in the world. I have had the privilege of working with Walter for almost two decades, and I have never failed to be impressed by his creativity and his extraordinary accomplishments. Walter is a physician and an internationally renowned scientist who has done some of science's most exciting work in several fields, including immunology, endocrinology, and aging. He is that rare combination: a man who not only has vision, but also has the training, intelligence, tools, and perseverance that help convert that vision into reality. He is a world-class scientist, but, like the best of scientists, he is also a humanist. Walter also has always been something of a maverick, and perhaps his extraordinary success is due to the fact that throughout his career he has been willing to challenge accepted scientific doctrine when his intuition told him to do so.

You may recall a time when doctors would dismissively tell patients who were suffering symptoms of illness with no obvious cause that their problems were "all in their heads." If today doctors are less prone to do that, if today doctors recognize that emotional (and physical) stress can profoundly affect every organ system in the body, and treat their patients accordingly, we have Walter in part to thank. Walter was one of the first researchers to establish what is now well known as the mind/body connection. He showed that our immune system, which keeps us well, and our endocrine system, which, among other things, controls how we respond to stress, are in constant communication, and that what happens to one invariably affects the other. As I think you will soon agree, Walter's greatest gift, and the thing that makes him a brilliant scientist, is his ability to intuitively sense, or see, connections that others might overlook.

I regard my work with Walter to be the culmination of a career devoted to doing pioneering work in new fields. After finishing medical school, I did my postgraduate training at Memorial Sloan-Kettering Cancer Research Institute, where I was one of the early researchers in the field of cancer chemotherapy and immunotherapy. Before chemotherapy and immuno-therapy, the only cancer treatment options were radia-tion and surgery, and these were ineffective against most cancers. After the Second World War, however, new drugs were developed that could actually sup-press the growth of tumor cells. These drugs provided the foundation for the sophisticated chemotherapy regimes that are used today, some with great success, to treat a wide range of cancers. I continued my re-search at Buffalo's Roswell Park Memorial Institute, the oldest cancer research center in the nation, and I later moved to Richmond to join the faculty of the Medical College of Virginia, Virginia Commonwealth University.

My interest in aging is a natural offshoot of my work in cancer research, because although cancer can strike anyone at any time, it is primarily a disease of aging. In other words, our risk of getting cancer increases significantly as we age. Cancer has reached epidemic proportions in the United States and other Western nations, and we have become so terrified of cancer that we do all kinds of things to try to escape it. We eat garlic cloves, pop vitamins by the handful, count fat grams, and consume large amounts of foods such as broccoli. There is certainly evidence that these measures may help, and I do not recommend that you abandon them. Indeed, I do some of these things my-self. But I have also reached the conclusion that an even more effective way of preventing cancer is by halting the physical deterioration that occurs in our bodies as we age. Those of us who are involved in aging research call this "remaining in the youthful state." Remaining in the youthful state does not mean that we do not get older. Time passes, no matter what we do. But it does mean that our bodies will not suffer the rapid decline that typifies how we age today. If we can remain in the youthful state, we can keep our bodies youthful and strong, and we can make ourselves less vulnerable to cancer and all other diseases as well. Melatonin, as we will explain, can help us take control of our bodies' aging clocks and remain in the youthful state.

The idea that aging is in any way controllable has been greeted with a certain amount of resistance on the part of the medical community. As a physician, I can tell you that most members of the medical profession are conservative, and that it can take years for a new idea, even for a very good new idea, to take hold and gain acceptance. History is replete with instances in which the medical establishment vigorously resisted new ideas that it later embraced wholeheartedly. A century ago, Louis Pasteur was ridiculed for suggesting that the tiny organisms he called microbes could actually cause disease. Similarly Ignaz Philipp Semmelweis in Vienna was persecuted because he said doctors ought to wash their hands before performing surgery. A half century ago, medical researchers who suggested that vitamin E might be a valuable treatment for heart disease were scoffed at. Today, heart patients are routinely given high doses of vitamin E after coronary bypass surgery because it has been shown to facilitate healing and prevent new blockages from occurring. A decade ago, two Australian medical researchers, Drs. Barry Marshall and Robin Warren, discovered that a bacterium called *H. pylori* causes most ulcers and that ulcers could be cured by treating them with antibiotics, not antacids. Their announcement was greeted with skepticism by nearly every organization of gastrointestinal specialists. Yet today, their therapy is the principal treatment for ulcers. I could go on, but I think that I've made my point: It can take a long time for new ideas to be integrated into the practice of medicine, and often patients suffer as a result of this acceptance lag.

Foreword

I am not recommending that we start using drugs and therapies that have not been adequately tested. What I am suggesting is that as a result of the resistance that the medical community so often shows to new treatments, many good ideas go untested, and, when it comes to funding research, too many truly imaginative and innovative investigators lose favor to those who pursue accepted doctrine. After practicing medicine and conducting research for several decades in an environment often resistant to change, I was determined to make it possible for scientists more easily to explore new, uncharted research paths. In 1980, I organized the Foundation Fund for Integrative Biomedical Research (FIBER), a group of scientists devoted to encouraging and funding innovative research in the field of aging. FIBER's goal was to promote interdisciplinary programs of research and provide seed money to scientists who had novel ideas to pursue, in order that they could get the recognition they needed to secure additional funding from traditional sources. Another of FIBER's goals was to foster a spirit of partnership and cooperation among scientists. Especially when funding is scarce, scientists who should be exchanging ideas become secretive and competitive, and this serves no one's interests, the public's least of all. FIBER's goal was to stimulate the free exchange of ideas among scientists, and we succeeded in this by holding a number of interesting conferences and promoting pivotal research directed at restoring and maintaining our youthful capacity.

Walter Pierpaoli is one of the innovative researchers who caught FIBER's attention, and we brought him to the United States to learn more about his remarkable work, and to introduce him to others in our scientific community for collaborative work.

The scientists whom I met in the course of my work with FIBER taught me no small amount about recent

Foreword

advances in aging research, and this inspired me to take up the study of a hormone called dehydroepi-androsterone, or DHEA for short, which has been shown to have some amazing properties. Among other things, it appears to protect against cancer and heart disease, improve memory, enhance mood, and improve sexual function in men. Although DHEA cannot control or reverse the aging process in the way melatonin does, it may prove to be another useful tool in maintaining our health and vigor. You will not be surprised to know that scientists have been seriously studying DHEA for more than thirty years, but the medical establishment is just beginning to take a hard look at this hormone. Since DHEA is available by prescription only, it will be some years before the public ever gets to experience its benefits.

And this is precisely why Walter and I decided to write this book at this time. We want to spread the word about melatonin, and how this hormone can help us maintain the youthful state. Our experiments on animals have convinced us of the power, value, and safety of melatonin, and we strongly believe that melatonin will have the same positive effect on humans. That is why we are taking it ourselves, and that is why we recommend it to our friends and loved ones. It is now time for the National Institute of Aging to initiate human studies on melatonin so we can learn more about this remarkable hormone.

We want to inform our colleagues, the pharmaceutical industry, and the FDA that much of the pathology of aging can be prevented. Congress and the public must be motivated to support research that recognizes certain aspects of aging as a syndrome that can be reversed or prevented.

I am seventy years old. To my surprise, I have suddenly become aware of my mortality. I can't afford to wait another thirty years. I don't want to see my creativity, my ability to enjoy the beauty of this earth, and the sensual joy of my body destroyed by a process that our research tells us is reversible and even preventable.

But we are not writing this book solely for personal reasons. We want to draw attention to the field of aging research in general. We feel we are doing this not a minute too soon. The population of the United States is rapidly aging. In just a few months, the first crop of baby boomers—who were born at the end of World War II—will turn fifty! In many ways, these "boomers" have led lives, indeed have approached life, in ways that set them apart from their parents and grandparents. For better or for worse, and we think generally for the better, members of the baby boom generation have managed to alter nearly every institution they have touched. Now, thanks to what we have discovered, we believe they can alter the institution of aging.

With the understanding that our wish can be a reality, Walter and I wish you good health and long life.

William Regelson, M.D.
Medical College of Virginia
Virginia Commonwealth University

PART ONE

Nature's Age-Reversing Hormone

CHAPTER 1

The Melatonin Miracle

Picture this.

It's your ninetieth birthday. You love your work, but you cancel your afternoon appointments in order to leave the office early to celebrate. You meet a friend at the club to play squash. Later, you head home to meet your spouse of sixty years. You know a special evening is in store for you—dinner at your favorite restaurant, a show, and then nightcaps or espresso at an after-hours jazz club. But the best is yet to come. You'll be spending the night at the same quaint but luxurious inn where you celebrated your fiftieth wedding anniversary. You've reserved the honeymoon suite, which features a Jacuzzi for two. Tomorrow will be a busy day as well. You promised your great-grandchildren that as soon as you finished your morning errands you would go roller blading with them in the park.

Does this sound fantastic? Do you have trouble believing that, when you are ninety years old, you can be working, living, and loving in much the same style and with much the same strength and vigor that you enjoyed at age thirty-five or forty?

Well, believe it.

Three decades of research and practice in the fields of immunology, oncology, biochemistry, and pathology have taught us that aging does not have to be the inevitable downward slide that we have grown resigned to facing. On the contrary, scientific evidence supports our belief that that discouraging vision of aging is a thing of the past.

This book does not present some futuristic vision of what your great-great-grandchildren's lives will be like a hundred years from now. This book is about what *your* life will be like when you are a hundred . . . and spending time (when you're not otherwise committed) with your great-great-grandchildren. This book is not a work of science fiction. Rather, it is a work of science. Thirty years of research have led us to an extraordinary discovery. Our discovery has not only changed the way we view aging, but will actually change the way people age. What we have learned will not merely add decades to your life, but will enable you to live those years in a strong, healthy, youthful body.

How do you view aging? If we ask you to close your eyes and picture yourself when you are "old," what image do you see? Chances are, you are picturing yourself bent and frail, and with passing years you imagine yourself growing weaker and progressively sicker, someone whose birthdays bring forth a flood of wistful reflections about the way things used to be, about the way *you* used to be. In short, you are picturing yourself as nostalgic for your lost youth, strength, and vitality.

It is time to discard this stereotype. Our discovery has taught us that the inexorable physical and mental decline that we have become all too accustomed to associating with aging need not occur. Thanks to what we have discovered, when you do reach your upper decades, you will not be sitting around bemoaning the loss of the health and vigor that you possessed in, say, your forties. You won't have any reason to do so, because you will not experience such a loss.

We are not suggesting that we can stop aging altogether. The years will continue to pass. So will the decades. But, as they do, the transitions from our sixties to seventies and eighties to nineties, and even to our hundreds, will be no more eventful than was our passage from our twenties to thirties to forties. Each passing year will not leave its stamp of decay. We will not fall apart and wither.

Our vision, of course, represents a radical departure from the traditional view of aging. For thousands of years, scientists have considered the process of aging to be as inevitable as the passage of time itself. Today, the aging process is synonymous with "senescence," a dismal, discouraging medical term used by doctors to describe the physical and mental deterioration that we have grown to accept as part and parcel of aging. According to the traditional view, aging is a downward spiral through a series of degenerative illnesses terminating in death. Physicians who care for aging patients tend to regard their patients as travelers on a one-way ticket, with each disease an unpleasant but unavoidable stop along the way. As one system breaks down after another, patients are referred to one specialist after another. Each specialist deals with his or her own small piece of the aging puzzle—trying to patch his piece up or replace it.

But these doctors, talented though they may be, do not view the puzzle, or the patient, as a whole. They aim to treat each symptom as it comes along (and, if they are worth their salt, they also aim to treat their patients with consideration and respect). But we have to say, with due respect in every direction, that their aim, to put it bluntly, is off the mark. We think that in addition to focusing on each symptom, we ought to be focusing on the underlying disease itself.

The underlying disease—indeed the ultimate disease—is aging. This book is about how to treat it.

We regard aging as the "ultimate disease" because, as the body ages, breakdown in bodily systems make us more susceptible to disease. Disease, in turn, causes the body to age. We believe that there is a way to intervene and break this aging → disease → aging cycle. When we do, we stave off both a major cause and a major effect of what we know as aging. In other words, when we treat aging itself—rather than its unfortunate symptoms—the frequency and effect of those symptoms will diminish.

This concept—revolutionary though it may seem—is the product of an evolution in our thinking that occurred as a result of the work we were doing in several fields, including immunology, pathology, and oncology. Neither of us is a gerontologist, and to be perfectly frank, we did not set out to test entrenched theories about how we age. Ironically, we think that it is precisely because our research was multidisciplinary that we developed a broader view of how we age, and were able to perceive connections that other researchers whose focus was more narrow did not see. Our work led us to the discovery of how and why we age, and, more importantly, how to control the process of aging itself.

We have identified the precise point in the brain that controls how we age—we call it the aging clock. We have determined how it works, and we have discovered the key to turning it back. In this book, we will describe in detail our research, which until this point has been published only in scholarly journals, revealing to the public at large how we discovered the aging clock, and how it functions. In the process, we will show you:

- How melatonin, a safe and inexpensive supplement that is already available at your neighborhood health food store, can turn back your aging clock, so that you can begin to slow down or even reverse the aging process, starting today.

- How you can extend your life span from the commonly projected seventy-five years to 120 years.
- How to reinvigorate your sex life (whether you are thirty, sixty, or ninety).
- How to revive your immune system so that you can live well and disease-free for a century or more.

Our research—which has been the focus of several international scientific conferences and which is described here in a nutshell—has taught us that the pineal gland, a pea-sized structure embedded deep within our brains, is the key to understanding, and controlling, how we age. The pineal gland is a part of the body that, until recent years, has been little studied but long revered. For example, the Hindus attached mystical importance to the pineal, referring to it as the body's "third eye," and, in a sense, that's what it is. The pineal gland, which contains pigment cells similar to those found in our eyes, is light-sensitive and reacts to periods of light and dark transmitted to it through our eyes. The pineal controls the body's biological clock, the internal mechanism that tells us when it's time to sleep and when it's time to wake up. Scientists refer to this daily sleep/wake cycle as our circadian rhythm. The pineal exerts its control through a hormone called melatonin, which it produces primarily at night when we are asleep.

But the pineal regulates more than our sleep patterns. It regulates the rhythms of life itself, and nowhere is this more apparent than in the animal kingdom, because the natural rhythms of animals' lives are not disrupted by alarm clocks or beepers. In spring, the pineal awakens lustful feelings, signaling to animals that it's the season to mate. As summer gives

7

way to autumn, the pineal signals to birds that it's time to migrate. The pineal gland even functions as an internal navigational system, keeping them on course as they traverse the globe. As winter approaches and daylight hours grow shorter, the pineal alerts animals that it's time to take shelter and hibernate. Months later, as days begin to lengthen, the pineal awakens them from winter's sleep.

In humans, the pineal's role is more subtle, but equally profound. We call the pineal the regulator of the regulators. It is the master gland that oversees the operation of our other glands, and, as a result, its influence is felt by every cell in our bodies. It helps us to maintain normal daily and seasonal hormone levels, and it oversees and superintends our growth and development from infancy through adulthood.

The pineal gland manufactures, and operates through, a hormone called melatonin. Melatonin is instrumental in establishing our daily rhythms, from infancy on. Expectant mothers pass melatonin to their developing babies through the placenta. Although infants don't manufacture their own supply of melatonin until their third or fourth day of life, melatonin is present in breast milk. Melatonin levels peak during childhood. During adolescence, melatonin levels drop, triggering a rise in other hormones, which in turn signal to the body that it is time to enter puberty. As we age, our melatonin levels continue to decrease, with the steepest decline occurring from about age fifty on. By age sixty, our pineal glands are producing half the amount of melatonin they did when we were twenty. Not so coincidentally, as melatonin levels drop, we begin to exhibit serious signs of aging.

For reasons that we will explain in more detail in later chapters, we believe that this drop in melatonin levels happens, and the downward spiral known as aging occurs, because the pineal gland—the aging clock—breaks down. When the aging clock begins to show signs of aging itself, it signals to other parts of the body that it is time for them to grow old too. What ensues is the all-too-familiar progressive, system-by-system breakdown that leads to disease, disability, and ultimately death. The aging process strikes some of us earlier than others. However, even the hardiest of the elderly eventually fall prey. Few of us manage to stay healthy and disease-free throughout our entire lives, and only a very lucky few manage to endure—let alone enjoy—our full living potential.

But our studies have shown us that it is possible to stop the aging process dead in its tracks. We have discovered how to "fix" or reset the aging clock so that we can remain vigorous and strong throughout our entire lives, and certainly well into our ninth and tenth decades. We also believe that we can fulfill our biological potential of living to be 120 years old and perhaps even longer than that. Although death is still inevitable, we are confident that we can forestall it, and not merely by adding dismal "golden years" that will be spent in bleak retirement villages, hospitals, and nursing homes. What we are talking about is years that are productive and enjoyable; years that any of us would rightly regard as among the best of our lives.

In order to understand how to fix the aging clock, you need to know why the clock breaks in the first place. We consider this in greater detail later on, but an overview is helpful here. We humans are highly socialized animals who, unlike our wilder counterparts, have evolved beyond the purely biological role that nature assigned us. We think and we dream, and we create and we pursue goals. As far as nature is concerned, however, we are here for one reason, and that is to reproduce. Consequently, when we reach a certain age and have, in theory or fact, reproduced, we are in nature's eyes expendable. Nature is not concerned with our lifetime dreams and ambitions that we have yet to fulfill. This may sound harsh, but it is, if you think about it, perfectly logical, and it is true not only for humans, but for other animal species as well. Salmon, for example, die shortly after they spawn. The female octopus literally starves herself to death after she reproduces. Male marsupial mice, related to the kangaroo, die after mating season. Of course, as you can see, we fare a lot better than these animals. Even after our reproductive years have passed, we still have quite a few left to go. But, clearly, we begin to wind down.

We wind down because the pineal gland—the aging clock—winds down. This happens because the pineal gland is constantly monitoring our bodies for signs of decline, such as a decline in the production of sex hormones. When the pineal detects that we are past our reproductive prime, it, in turn, begins to break or slow down, signaling our bodies that it is time to age. We have identified a simple way to "trick" the pineal gland into thinking that we are still young and vigorous. We have found a way to halt and even reverse the process that we have been taught to believe is normal aging.

Melatonin is the key to "resetting" the clock. In animal studies at Dr. Pierpaoli's Biancalana-Masera Foundation for the Aged in Ancona, Italy, we have shown that melatonin supplements, given at the right time, can stop and reverse the aging process. In one early study, we gave one group of old mice melatonin in their night drinking water, and compared their physical characteristics and behavior to an identical group of mice who did not get melatonin. Six months later, the untreated mice continued to show signs of aging —they developed patchy bald spots, they grew shriveled, they lost neuromuscular coordination, they lost immune and thyroid responsiveness, and they slowed down until they all eventually died of cancer, which is the typical pattern of aging and death for this particular breed of mice. The melatonin-treated mice experienced a dramatically different fate. To our astonishment, they seemed to "grow young," practically overnight. Their fur grew thick and lustrous, their bodies grew slim and supple, and their youthful motor activity returned. Tests showed that their immunity against disease had vastly improved. Their energy levels increased, and much to our amazement, their sexual vigor was restored. What's even more exciting is that the melatonin mice lived on average 30 percent longer than the untreated mice, which in human terms is a gain of about twenty to twenty-five years. Even more astounding was the fact that the melatonin mice did not succumb to the deadly cancer that invariably affects their breed.

Since our early work, we have performed other studies that even more dramatically identify the pineal gland as the body's aging clock and melatonin as its messenger. In a series of groundbreaking studies that attracted the attention of the international scientific community, we transplanted pineal glands from young animals into old animals. We were excited to find that the old animals with the young pineal glands began to rejuvenate. They looked, and also acted, like young animals. We then transplanted pineal glands from old animals into young animals. The young animals with the old pineals began to age rapidly—they looked and acted like old animals, and they died well before their time. Later in the book, we will talk more about these experiments and what they can teach us about the aging process.

Based on thirty years of research and experimentation, we are convinced that melatonin is the key to health and longevity. We take it ourselves, and so do the people in our lab. We recommend it to our families and loved ones. Dr. Pierpaoli has given melatonin to Emmy, his former mother-in-law, since 1984, when she was seventy-four, to help stave off the early symptoms of Parkinson's disease, a common neurological disease among the elderly that can cause tremors and can make it difficult to perform such simple tasks as holding a teacup. Now, ten years later, she is sharp, active, and free of Parkinson's symptoms. We believe this is related to her melatonin treatments. We should also add that her skin is as smooth and practically wrinkle-free as it was a decade ago. As word got out about our experiences with melatonin, and as more experiments began to document melatonin's remarkable effects, many other researchers in the field of aging began to take melatonin as well. From these and other studies that we will discuss later in the book, we have determined that the aging process can be postponed, and even reversed, simply by restoring melatonin to youthful levels.

Although melatonin is something that most people have not heard of before, the theory of hormone replacement is not new or untried. On the contrary, today, millions of women, after menopause, routinely take hormone-replacement therapy to restore their estrogen to more youthful levels. The theory here is very similar. We recommend that when melatonin levels naturally begin to decline (usually around age forty-five), people should begin to take melatonin supplements in order to boost their levels back to what they were at age twenty. We want to stress that we are not telling people to take melatonin indiscriminately. We recommend doses that are considerably more conservative than what is usually found in commercial melatonin supplements. In Chapter 14 "How to Take Melatonin: The Right Dosages," we will tell you how to take melatonin safely and effectively, and how to determine the dosage that is right for you. We believe that, armed with the information about the mechanics of aging and the role that the pineal gland and melatonin play in the process, you will be able to do simple things that will enable you to turn back the hands of time and postpone the aging process.

Let us be clear on something: Melatonin is neither a panacea nor a "happy pill" that will provide quick fixes or superficial results. Based on what we know about melatonin, its beneficial effects will be felt gradually, over time. For obvious reasons, when we think about aging, we are inclined to focus on its more superficial, outward manifestations. We notice that we are getting older when, for example, our hair begins to turn gray, when we notice our first wrinkles, or when we have to be fitted for our first pair of bifocals. But as alarming as we may find those outward symbols of aging, what is happening inside our bodies is far more subtle and insidious. What we are suggesting is that the way to approach aging is to address the inward conditions that give rise to various outward symptoms. Only by curing aging from the inside out, so to speak, will we truly achieve an effective means of reversing the outward signs of aging.

Aging is actually the loss of the body's ability to adapt to its environment. Our bodies are constantly forced to respond to various stresses and stimuli, such as adjusting to a temperature change, fighting off a virus, or even just knowing when it's time to sleep and wake. Think of your body as a rubber band. When we're young and strong, our bodies can easily bounce back from the force of these stresses, but, as we age, we increasingly lose our ability to rapidly adapt to new situations—in short, we lose our resiliency. Like an old, worn-out rubber band, it takes us longer and longer to bounce back. We can't take the cold (or the heat) as well as we once could. When we get a virus we get sicker and take longer to recuperate. We have trouble falling asleep. Melatonin can restore the normal balance and durability that we lose as we age. It can keep us resilient, and it is that resiliency that keeps us young.

MELATONIN THE MIRACLE

Melatonin is a potent age-reversing compound, and we are confident that melatonin's primary benefit is in its ability to prevent disease by preventing the downward spiral that leads to illness. Scientists in laboratories all over the world are also investigating the role of melatonin in treating specific ailments. For example:

- Researchers at Tulane University School of Medicine in New Orleans have shown that melatonin can inhibit the growth of human breast cancer cells. Oncologists in Milan have actually been using melatonin to treat cancer patients in conjunction with traditional chemotherapy and immunotherapy. They have reported that melatonin-treated patients showed tumor regression and lived longer with fewer side effects than those who did not receive melatonin.
- Several studies have shown that melatonin is a safe, effective treatment for insomnia. Unlike other sleeping pills that disrupt REM (dream) sleep, melatonin actually restores normal sleeping and dreaming patterns.
- Melatonin is an excellent cure for jet lag. Melatonin pills taken at the right time can help restore normal sleep/wake cycles that are disrupted by flying across time zones.

- Melatonin may help prevent heart disease, the number one killer of men and women in the United States and many other Western countries. Studies show that melatonin can lower blood cholesterol levels in people who have high cholesterol, helping to control a major risk factor for heart attack and stroke.

All of these, and other exciting applications for what is truly the miracle hormone of our lifetimes, will be covered in later chapters of this book.

WHY THIS BOOK, WHY US, WHY NOW?

We are writing this book for several reasons. First, we're excited about our research and its potential for improving people's lives and lifestyles. We want to share it with others, and feel it is important that we do so now, not in ten or twenty years. Some of our more conservative colleagues may accuse us of jumping the gun and reporting our findings prematurely, before melatonin has undergone a battery of "official" tests, including the rigors of human clinical studies. Frankly, by the time melatonin (which, to repeat, is already available over the counter) is thoroughly researched and scrutinized by every official panel, time will have run out for most of us.

Science can (by necessity) move at a painfully slow pace, especially in countries such as the United States, where decades may pass before an idea becomes mainstream. The link between diet and cancer and diet and heart disease are good examples. If you're middle-aged, like we are, you don't have the luxury of a twenty-year wait. As of this writing, Walter is a youthful sixty who has recently embarked on a second marriage, and Bill is a remarkable seventy with

15

an equally remarkable wife, six grown children, and six grandchildren. We both have a lot to live for: We lead full, extremely vigorous, and interesting lives that we love, and we want to continue to do so for as long as possible. If there is something that we can do today to reverse the aging process, and to push our scientific understanding of aging, we want to do it right now. We are not willing to wait the two or three decades that it will take before melatonin gets the official nod, and we don't think that it is fair to ask the public to wait either.

Besides, there are reasons to believe that with melatonin in particular, there is a need to go public in order to ensure that melatonin will receive all the attention that it rightfully deserves from the scientific community. We readily concede that we are only just beginning to unravel the mysteries of melatonin, and its effect on the aging process. But, given melatonin's promise as an age-reversing agent—and one that may prove to be an effective treatment for cancer and other life-threatening ailments—more research is desperately needed. This will only happen if the public demands it. Because melatonin occurs naturally (like vitamin C), it can't be patented. Therefore, drug companies have little incentive to spend the hundreds of millions of dollars required to study melatonin. That leaves it in the hands of government to fund studies of melatonin—but will it? As government slashes its support for scientific research, researchers are already scrambling for funds. Many good, solid ideas will never be investigated—and tragically, as a result many lives will be lost—due to lack of funding. We hope to create a groundswell of interest in melatonin in order to encourage further scientific melatonin research.

Much of the research that currently does get government and private funding deals with the diseases of aging, but not the aging process itself. Compared to the great leaps made in other branches of science, such as theoretical physics, biology is still in the Stone Age. We have still not found cures for the same diseases that plagued us hundreds of years ago, and we are helpless when faced with new plagues. We have made great strides in the prolongation of life, but that is primarily due to better diet, improved hygiene and the use of antibiotics or vaccines, not to a better understanding of basic biology, which we believe is the true key to fighting disease. If we intervene and reverse the aging process, we can thereby prevent many diseases from occurring in the first place. Although we don't want to divert precious money from research that may lead to valuable treatments for people who are already sick, we do believe that, in the long run, more people will benefit from our preventive approach.

We are also concerned that greed—sometimes disguised as a misguided desire to "protect" the public —will prevail over the right of the public to know. There are rumors that some pharmaceutical companies, seeking to profit by marketing melatonin as a sleeping pill or other type of drug, are lobbying to convince the Food and Drug Administration to make melatonin available by prescription only. We strongly believe that this would be a terrible mistake. Something as safe and as important to our health and well-being as melatonin should remain inexpensive and easily available to the public. It should be so for everyone —not just for the select few who can get prescriptions, or who can afford to pay the steep price tag typical of today's newly approved drugs. Naturally, there are also legitimate questions being raised concerning such important issues as quality control, particularly with regard to melatonin products derived from animals. However, there is a better solution to the problem of quality control than simply pulling melatonin off the market. For the purposes of safety, hygiene, and consistency, we recommend using a synthetic form of melatonin. There are several synthetic brands already available, and we predict, as the demand for melatonin increases, there will be more, and that they will be produced by the same reputable companies that market other high-quality supplements.

Finally, and in many respects most importantly, we are writing this book to change your expectations about how you can and should age. If our society continues to be complacent about aging, if we don't challenge the conventional wisdom that aging is an inevitable downward spiral, we will be cheating ourselves out of decades of life—and not just life in an impaired physical state, but life as we cherish it today: in a strong, healthy, youthful body.

In Part One of this book, we will focus on the scientific journey that led to the discovery of the aging clock. That odyssey will take readers around the world—from Switzerland to Italy to Russia—to a variety of different laboratories where Walter did his groundbreaking experiments. Readers will learn about the remarkable pineal gland, and how it controls your every action. Readers will also come to learn all that is so far known about melatonin, and how it can literally change your life.

Life, of course, is ultimately what our book is all about. We hope that readers will receive the Melatonin Miracle as the celebration of life we intend it to be, and that it will encourage and inspire each and everyone to take control of their own destinies and accept our life-affirming message: It is possible to live longer than you ever imagined. What is more important, it is possible to live those extra decades with the same level of health and vigor that we associate with our youth and middle age.

CHAPTER 2

Pierpaoli's Story: First Clues in the Hunt for the Aging Clock

*"It is impossible for anyone to begin to learn
what he believes he already knows."*

—Epictetus (c. a.d. 55–c. 135)

When I explain to people about the aging clock and the role that the pineal gland plays in regulating our body systems, I find that they are able to catch on very quickly if I start with an analogy. Imagine a symphony orchestra. In one section are the string instruments, in another area are the woodwinds, and in another are the brass horns, and so forth. If you play the violin, you sit among the other violinists and you play your part. If you play the clarinet, you sit among the other clarinetists and you play your part. Since your parts are very different, they might seem to be totally unrelated and independent of one another. But of course, we know that this is not true. All we have to do is step back and stand in the position of the conductor to see that the performance of each orchestra section is interdependent upon the others, and that when the musicians follow the directions of the conductor, they produce beautiful music.

We have discovered that the pineal gland is to our bodies what the conductor is to the orchestra. The job of the pineal gland is to regulate and harmonize the functioning of a number of our bodily systems. One of these systems is our endocrine system, which is made up of many glands that produce the hormones that control our growth from childhood to adulthood. They also control our sexual development. Another of these systems is the immune system, which protects us against disease. In its capacity as the regulator of these systems, the pineal also functions as the body's aging clock. When the pineal begins to run down, so do all the other systems under its control. To return to our analogy, it is as if the orchestra conductor has become too tired to lead the orchestra. The musicians become disorganized and unable to play in concert. The performance breaks down and finally stops altogether.

When I explain the theory of the aging clock in these terms, listeners say, "Aha! That makes sense." Of course it does make perfect sense that a body as complex as ours, in which literally thousands of activities are taking place simultaneously, would require some kind of central regulator to monitor these activities, to keep them functioning in harmony with one another and with the outside world, and to tell them when to start and when to stop. Such is the nature of hindsight. Yet, when I began my career as a scientist more than thirty years ago, the mere suggestion of the existence of some kind of centralized regulator, or aging clock, would have been dismissed as utterly ridiculous. The prevailing wisdom at the time was that each of the body's systems operated independently, and whole schools of thought grew up around one particular organ system or another. You were either a "heart man," or a "bone man" or an "endocrine man." (I use the word "man" advisedly, because back then there were very few women in the field of medicine.) Gerontologists, who specialize in the study of aging, generally believed that aging occurred in a random fashion in individual cells, and that gradually, as more and more cells wore out, the body aged and died. (To employ our orchestra analogy again, it would be as if individual musicians decided that they were getting tired, threw down their instruments, and stalked off the stage. As more and more followed suit, the music would peter out and eventually stop altogether.) The notion that this cellular burnout could have been triggered or governed by a centralized regulator, a conductor, would have been considered absurd. If, back then, a colleague or student had presented such a theory to me, I, too, would probably have dismissed them and their idea as preposterous.

Discovering the aging clock required a radical shift in my thinking and my focus. It required that I, too, step back and put myself in the position of the orchestra conductor and take a wide-angle look at the entire body and not just focus on one or two of its seemingly separate systems. It also required, quite literally, many thousands of hours in my laboratories over three decades, countless frustrations, and the occasional revelation that moved my work forward. But such is the nature of science.

If I have been successful as a scientist, I attribute that success in large part to my training—or, to be more accurate, my *cross*-training. I am neither a gerontologist nor a pinealogist (someone who has devoted his career to the study of the pineal gland). I prefer to call myself a generalist, because, throughout my career, I have tried very hard not to become confined to any small corner of medicine. I have always feared that overspecialization would lead to intellectual isola-

21

tion, which for a scientist can be deadly. It's of critical importance to keep abreast of developments in all fields, and to try to understand how they relate to your own area of interest. Very often an important finding in one area of science can profoundly affect another.

In keeping with my philosophy, I have always made a special point to straddle several different scientific fields. I am a medical doctor with special training in biochemistry and pathology, and I hold a Ph.D. in immunology. A pathologist studies the disease process to develop treatments and cures. Although pathology is a noble vocation, for me it was never enough. I always felt that the real challenge was to prevent illness from occurring in the first place. I could not help but feel that by the time a patient was actually sick, the battle was half lost. This led me to the study of immunology because, when we do get sick, it is due to a malfunction in our immune system. The immune system is the body's first line of defense against disease. It operates as a surveillance system, continuously monitoring the body for the presence of viruses, bacteria, and other foreign invaders. The immune system is actually a highly complex army of cells that protect the body against viruses, bacteria, and other foreign invaders, including some forms of cancer cells. If our immune systems are basically healthy and strong, then they will keep us healthy. But if our immune systems weaken, they become less able to fend off viral and bacterial infections, or they may be unable to distinguish between normal and abnormal cells and some forms of cancer may result. Thus, it has always seemed to me that if we could figure out how to keep the immune system functioning properly, we would be able to keep many of our most destructive illnesses at bay. Such an achievement is, to my way of thinking, the essence of true preventative medicine.

In addition to being a pathologist and immunologist,

Nature's Age-Reversing Hormone

I am a physician and I was trained to work with patients. This has affected the way that I do my research. It so happens that many scientific researchers, generally those who are not physicians, conduct their research by observing cells in a test tube. This is known as in vitro experimentation. It is not the methodology I prefer. In my opinion, and it is no doubt colored by experience treating patients, there is a real difference between working in vitro and working in vivo, that is, with living, breathing, feeling, flesh-and-blood creatures. Thus, although I chose a career in research, I still prefer to work with animal models instead of isolated cells. Animal experiments are far more time-consuming and trickier to perform than test tube studies, yet there is no better way to do science. As a physician, I was taught to look at the whole patient, not to focus solely on the disease. If you really want to know how a molecule reacts in the body, or how one bodily system interacts with another, you have to observe the reaction in a working body. To me it is unthinkable that one could find the cause of aging simply by observing cells in a petri dish.

I work with mice. I sometimes joke that I am a "mouse doctor," because, over the past thirty years, I have worked with literally thousands of mice. I think it is fair to say that I know all there is to know about mice. Now, this is not as odd or funny as it may sound, because mice, in fact, provide a wonderful model for the study of human disease. These tiny creatures fall prey to the same diseases as we do, and in mice the pathology of these diseases—that is, the way the illnesses play out in their bodies—is nearly identical to the pathology of these diseases in humans. Scientists know this very well. That is why mice are used for so much of today's medical research, whether it is research to test a new cancer drug or to develop a vaccine against HIV.

Mice are also subject to the same basic biological rhythms as humans. Frankly, if I had been working only with cells in a test tube, I would have missed several vital clues that could only have come from observing the behavior of living beings subject to the same life cycles that we are. But I'm jumping ahead. I will get to all that later in the story.

I began my work as a researcher in the field of immunology in the 1960s. To me, being an immunologist in that era was like being an explorer in the days of Columbus or Vasco da Gama, two men who connected the Old World to the New and in doing so changed the course of history. In immunology, new frontiers were being forged almost daily. Scientists were just beginning to unravel the mysteries of the immune system. They were learning how immune cells produced antibodies specifically tailored to identify and ward off enemy antigens, agents that the body deems to be dangerous. They were also learning how immune cells called lymphocytes attack viruses, bacteria, and any foreign substances the body does not identify as its own. Immunologists were also desperately trying to learn how to turn off the immune system so that they could transplant organs, such as hearts and kidneys, without the recipient's body rejecting them.

CONNECTING THE BODY AND THE MIND

I was beginning my journey in a field that was on the brink of major upheavals and new discoveries, and often I found that I was navigating through uncharted and, at times, hostile waters. For example, today the term "mind/body connection" is commonplace. We take for granted that the mind and the rest of the body are inextricably linked and that each has a profound effect on the other. Today, we know that physical health cannot be separated from our feelings and emotions. For example, science has taught us that extreme stress can actually weaken the ability of our immune system to fight disease. We know that the hormones produced when we are under severe or sustained physical or emotional stress can actually destroy our body's disease-fighting cells, lessening our resistance to bacteria, viruses, and cancer-causing agents, when they invade our bodies. We know that when a mouse with a cancerous tumor is put on a constantly rotating platform—a situation that is extremely stressful for the mouse—the stress will actually trigger faster tumor growth. We know that during the time that marathon runners are training for a big race, they are more vulnerable to colds and flu. We also know that people who are emotionally depressed experience a depressed immune response. We also know that there are some diseases, such as chronic fatigue syndrome, that are believed to have psychological and physical origins.

Ancient healers and Native American shamans or medicine men seem to have intuitively understood the link between physical and emotional health, and they often attributed illness of the body to an underlying illness of the psyche or the soul. But in the 1960s many thoughtful people—mainstream scientists included—would have dismissed as pure hokum the mind/body connections that today are widely recognized as true. You have to understand that immunologists of that not-so-distant era considered the immune system to be a fortress unto itself. The immune system was believed to be a separate army, marching to the beat of its own drum, following marching orders that were separate and distinct from those governing other body systems. It would have been ridiculous even to suggest that the hormones produced by another body system could have any impact on the insulated immune system.

That is how the immunologists viewed the world. Then there were the endocrinologists. Endocrinologists of that era also considered "their system," the endocrine system, to be an island unto *itself*. They could not imagine that their glands, which produce the hormones that govern growth and sexual development, and that influence how we react to stress, could possibly affect the immune system. But of course, we now know that these two seemingly separate systems in fact are in constant communication with each other, and cannot even function without each other's input. I'll explain more about this interrelationship as we progress, and how this concept actually led to the discovery of the critical role of the pineal gland as the "regulator" of many of our bodily activities. First you need to know a bit about the endocrine system and the hormones which it produces and how this relates to the clock which governs aging.

A hormone is a chemical messenger that tells the cells of the body what to do and when to do it. Hormones control virtually every function in the body, and, in particular, they control growth, sexual development, and aging. When you think of hormones, you probably think of sex, and for good reason. The sex organs are major players in this endocrine system, and the hormones that they produce are what make us sexual beings. Estrogen, which is produced in the female's ovaries, is what gives women their "feminine" characteristics: It makes their skin soft, their breasts full, and along with other hormones controls their monthly menstrual cycle. Testosterone, which is produced in the male testes, is what gives men their "maleness": It makes hair grow on their face and bodies, it makes their voices deepen at puberty, and it is instrumental in the production of sperm. When we touch, cuddle, kiss, and make love, each of these actions triggers our glands to release hormones that cause us to become aroused and enjoy our sexuality.

Hormones are involved in much of the aging process, from childhood through old age. Puberty is an event that is triggered by a dramatic rise in the levels of sex hormones. Menopause, which marks the passage from youth to middle age in women, occurs because the production of estrogen begins to drop precipitously. Although males don't experience menopause per se, they do experience a subtle shift in hormone levels as they age. There are many glands in the endocrine system. You've probably heard of the pituitary gland, which is sometimes called the master gland because it makes hormones that control other glands. It is located deep inside the brain, and, among other things, produces the growth hormone that controls how children grow. If children don't get enough growth hormone, their growth will be stunted. Another neuroendocrine center, the hypothalamus, which is located at the base of the brain, actually exerts some control over the pituitary gland. It also helps regulate such essential body functions as the sensation of hunger and thirst. Yet another endocrine gland, the thyroid, which sits at the base of the neck, secretes hormones that control metabolism, the way the body burns oxygen to carry out much of its other activities. If you don't make enough thyroid hormone, you will feel sluggish, you will have trouble maintaining your body temperature, you will gain weight, and every major system in your body will be slowed down. The adrenal glands, located atop the kidneys, produce stress hormones, that is, the hormones that are pumped out when we are under duress. Adrenaline, produced by the adrenals, is known as the "flight-or-fight" hormone because it provides a burst of energy that enables the body to respond quickly to stressful situations. The adrenal glands also produce sex hormones.

It may appear as if the endocrine system, which produces this array of hormones, and the immune system, with its army of disease-fighting cells, work independently of each other. But the links are there. Like the many different-looking and sounding instruments in the orchestra, these systems work in concert. Mainstream science has come around to accepting their interdependency. I like to think that I was fortunate enough to see this relationship early, and was something of a pioneer in making these connections. It was my work in this field that started me on the road that led to the discovery of the pineal's role as the orchestra leader, and ultimately, as the aging clock. It was through these connections that I learned how we age, and how to reverse the aging process. Against this backdrop, I will describe the twists and turns that I encountered along the way.

People who are not scientists rarely get a behind-the-scenes look at what is really involved in making a scientific breakthrough. You may read about major discoveries, after the fact, in the science section of your local newspaper, but these articles tend to focus on the findings and rarely report about the arduous, painstaking work that led to the discovery. I think this is a shame, not merely because I believe scientists deserve credit for working hard, but because the scientific journey can sometimes be every bit as interesting as the destination itself. To prove my point, I am going to devote the next few pages to giving you a glimpse of what it's like to be a scientist in search of an answer, how one clue sometimes connects to another, and how, if the correct questions are asked, important answers may be revealed.

Clue Number 1:
The Thymus and the "Aging" Mice

My hunt for the aging clock began more than thirty years ago, when, after studying the results of a scientific experiment performed by a brilliant colleague of mine, I found myself haunted by something I had seen. In order to understand this sensation, and how it set me on the trail of the aging clock, I need to give you a bit of background information.

Medical history is full of cases in which organs and glands, long dismissed as vestigial and unnecessary, have later been found to be of extreme importance. A case in point is the pineal gland, which is now known as the all-important regulator of the regulators. Until the past few decades, however, it was considered to be totally unnecessary. The thymus, a pinkish gray gland that sits behind the breastbone, is yet another gland that was once considered to be useless at best, and perhaps even dangerous. For centuries, a great deal of mystery and myth has surrounded the thymus. The thymus weighs about one half ounce at birth and doubles in size by puberty. Then, for reasons unknown, it begins to shrink and disappear, until it is gradually replaced by fatty tissue in adults. Until the 1960s, the thymus (like the pineal) had been considered an utterly useless gland. In fact, having a large thymus was considered a serious threat to health.

In the 1960s, two great scientists, the late Branislav D. Jankovic, of Belgrade, a close friend of mine, and Jacques Miller, of Australia, discovered that the thymus is neither useless nor dangerous. On the contrary, they found that this gland plays a critical role in immunity. In separate experiments, these scientists removed the thymus from newborn mice and rats. The effect was most dramatic: The mice never developed a

29

normal immune system. These thymus-less mice could not make antibodies, the cells that fight against disease. Not surprisingly, they died prematurely.

In light of what we today know about the thymus, these findings make perfect sense. Thanks to Jankovic and Miller, science has figured out that the thymus is filled with T lymphocytes, or T cells, important immune cells that fight against infection. Without T cells, you would die. This is precisely what happens to AIDS patients, because the HIV virus targets and destroys their T cells, leaving them vulnerable to infection. In children, T cells migrate from the bone marrow, where they are manufactured, to the thymus, where they mature and are stored, until they are called into action to defend against invading organisms. Without a thymus, the immune system cannot develop and mature properly.

In my own laboratory, when I removed the thymus from newborn mice, I was struck by the fact that the mice who had their thymuses removed looked not only sick, but, at least to my pathologist's eyes, they actually looked worn and wasted. Their coats were ragged, their muscles were atrophied. They looked like little, shriveled-up old men. I could not shake the feeling that these mice had not only fallen prey to disease, but had actually "aged," albeit without actually growing old.

I kept turning a question over in my mind: What could have caused the mice to age so rapidly? Could the thymus, now shown to play an important role in keeping us well, also play some role in aging? Might the thymus somehow be connected to the endocrine glands that control growth and aging? Was there a link between the thymus and pituitary gland? The sex glands? I devised an experiment to see if the thymus was somehow "talking" to these other glands.

Hypothesis: The Thymus "Talks" to the Pituitary

The pituitary gland is instrumental in how we grow and mature, from infancy through old age. As we noted earlier, it secretes growth hormone, which controls how children develop, and it exercises control over other glands that produce sex hormones.

We've seen that removal of the thymus gland in young mice caused the mice to rapidly "grow up," as well as grow sick. This made me wonder whether there was some connection between the immune system—which fights disease—and the endocrine system—which regulates how our bodies grow and age. I considered the possibility that the pituitary gland, which is essential for normal growth and sexual development, could somehow affect the thymus, and vice versa, so I devised some experiments to test my theory.

In the first experiment, I injected young adult mice with a serum that would prevent their pituitary glands from secreting any hormones. In other words, it would be as if these animals did not have a pituitary gland at all. As might be expected, these animals did not grow normally. They experienced weight loss, and a wasting disease similar to what I had seen in the mice without a thymus. Not only that, their thymuses shrunk or disappeared completely. Now, remember, the thymus is part of the immune system, the system that was supposed to be a "fortress unto itself." But my experiment showed that the functioning of the immune system was also affected by the pituitary gland, which controls growth and sexual development. Now it was time to turn the question around and see what would happen to the pituitary if I removed the thymus. In other words, I had shown that the pituitary spoke to the thymus. Now I had to see whether the thymus talked back to the pituitary.

31

In my second experiment, I removed the thymus glands from newborn mice and then examined the pituitary glands of these mice at various ages. Once again, the loss of the thymus resulted in the same wasting syndrome, and again I was struck by how much the mice resembled little old men. I also found that their production of hormones was thrown completely out of whack. When I looked at the pituitary glands of these mice, I could understand why hormone production had gone so awry. At the site in the pituitary glands where growth hormone is produced, there were gross abnormalities in the cells. The pituitaries could no longer produce the correct amount of growth hormone. No wonder the mice had matured so abnormally!

From these studies, I concluded that the thymus and the pituitary did talk to each other and were dependent on each other, and that neither a mouse (nor a human being) could grow normally unless both of these glands were intact and in constant communication. The bridge had been made: The thymus, which is part of the immune system, is essential for the proper functioning of the pituitary, which is part of the endocrine system; the reverse is also true.

These findings led me to ask yet another question. If removing the thymus could have such an adverse effect on the pituitary, and somehow accelerate aging, is the thymus, then, involved in the aging process itself? Do we age because our thymus gland tells us to age? I was not the only scientist pondering this question. Some researchers had begun to suspect that the thymus might even be the point in the body that controls aging; the so-called aging clock. Frankly, I had my doubts about this. I did believe that the thymus was one important player in aging, but that there had to be a larger explanation. I needed to devise further experiments to test my theory.

Hypothesis: The Thymus Isn't the Aging Clock

I, in addition to some other scientists, began to suspect that there was a "switch" somewhere in the body that controls how and when we age. We had begun calling it the "aging clock." We just did not know where it was or what it was. Some of my colleagues believed that it was the thymus, the gland behind the breastbone that stores our disease-fighting T cells, but I had a hunch that the thymus was not the answer.

My next group of experiments involved mice who had their thymus glands removed at birth. I had performed many experiments on mice without thymus glands. I knew from these experiments that if I transplanted a thymus from a normal mouse into a mouse without a thymus I could restore normal immune function and the mouse would then live out its normal life span. It would not get sick and grow old before its time. Some scientists believed that the thymus was responsible for maintaining life span. I believed, however, that the normal life span was shortened in these mice, not because the thymus, on its own, determined or could extend life span, but because its removal impaired immune function.

To test my theory, I needed to prove that if mice without thymus glands could somehow stay healthy, then they could also live out their normal life span. This would prove that these mice were dying young because they were getting sick due to their poor immune function, not because they lacked a thymus. In order to keep these mice healthy, I needed to raise them under completely sterile conditions, isolated from exposure to harmful viruses or bacteria. You probably have heard of children who are born with such seriously impaired immune systems that their very survival depends on their being kept in a sterile environment so they are not exposed to disease-causing organisms. Even a simple cold virus, which a healthy child could shake off in a few days, can be lethal to these immune-deficient children. They have been called "bubble" children because they must live in sealed, sterile, plastic bubble-like structures that protect them from a germ-filled world. Tragically, even their own parents cannot touch them or hug them without layers of protective garb. I needed to create a similar environment for my immune-impaired mice. I knew that Ciba-Geigy, a Swiss pharmaceutical company, had a unique laboratory in which they raised animals in a totally germ-free environment similar to the bubble. I made arrangements to use the laboratory's unique facilities.

We live in a world of germs. They outnumber us by the hundreds of billions. Avoiding them is a true art. My experiment required the utmost precision and attention to detail. Everything—and everybody—that came in contact with these mice had to be scrupulously clean. We took extreme measures to maintain sterile conditions. The first germ-free mice were delivered by cesarean section, so that they would not be contaminated by germs in the birth canal. This was a very delicate procedure performed under a special surgical microscope, requiring the use of tiny instruments. What added to the challenge was that in order to maintain a sterile environment, I had to wear special gloves and work through the curtain of an isolator that made it even more difficult to maneuver the delicate surgical instruments. I quite literally lived at the laboratory during this experiment, carefully monitoring the mice, day and night.

The results proved well worth the effort. Under these pristine conditions, there was no difference between the life span of the mice without thymus glands and mice that had thymuses. In other words, in natural conditions in the outside world, the mice without thymus glands had been dying young from disease due to poor immune response, not because the thymus was instrumental in controlling life span.

This experiment conclusively proved that the thymus was not controlling life span, and that the thymus was not the aging clock. But if the thymus was not the aging clock, what was? Was it another gland? Was it somewhere in the brain or somewhere else? Was it something I hadn't even considered?

Hypothesis: Sex Is Linked to Immunity

As part of my research on growth and aging, I performed many more experiments, and each experiment identified more links between the immune system and the hormones involved in growth and sexual development. I learned that the thymus was connected to the adrenal glands. The adrenal glands are located on top of the kidneys and, among other things, produce sex hormones. When an animal does not have a thymus gland it does not produce enough of these sex hormones, and does not develop properly. An abnormally low level of sex hormones results in stunted growth, and a strange, shriveled appearance.

I found another interesting link, this one between the thyroid gland, which is located at the base of the neck, and the thymus. When an animal did not have a thymus, it did not produce the right amount of thyroid hormone. Thyroid hormone is very important for normal immune function, and it is also very important for normal growth. If a baby is born with an underactive thyroid, severe mental retardation can result if the problem is not corrected.

These findings encouraged me to pursue the link between immunity and growth. I wanted to learn precisely how the immune system was involved in aging.

Other experiments performed with my colleague and friend Nicola Fabris, involved dwarf mice, yet another breed of mouse with a genetic flaw, one that prevents them from growing to normal size. In addition to their small stature, they have severe hormonal and immunological irregularities. Their thymus glands are very small, they are vulnerable to disease, they age quickly, and show the same wasting syndrome as mice without a thymus. Their levels for many critical hormones, including growth hormone, are significantly lower than those of normal mice. Scientists like myself have spent a great deal of time trying to correct the abnormalities in dwarf mice, and by doing so, have learned more about the action of various hormones.

In the first experiment, the connection between immunity and growth became even more apparent. We injected dwarf mice with growth hormone, which is produced by the pituitary. We were astonished to see that their thymus glands grew larger, and their immune systems grew stronger. The mice went on to live a much longer life than usual for dwarf mice. This provided yet more evidence of a direct line of communication between immunity and growth.

My second experiment with dwarf mice was simple, but it yielded some very interesting results. We injected mature lymphocytes (immune cells) from normal mice into dwarf mice. Their immune systems were revived, but what was more surprising was that these mice actually aged better than the untreated dwarf mice. They seemed to grow up more like normal mice. This was further evidence that the cells from the immune system were somehow "talking" to the endocrine system, influencing not only immunity, but growth patterns as well.

A definite and unmistakable pattern was emerging. Clearly, the glands involved in growth and sexual development—the pituitary, the adrenals, the thyroid, and perhaps others—were all communicating with one another—and they were also communicating with the thymus and the immune system. Nature had hooked the glands responsible for growth, reproduction, and immunity into one interdependent network. I didn't know why nature had done this, but I assumed it was for a good reason. If these activities are linked, I thought, perhaps there was some central regulator watching over them. This bit of deduction would later help me to formulate the theory that would lead to the discovery of the aging clock.

The orchestra pit was beginning to fill up with players, but where was the conductor?

Something in the Brain

As I continued my work in this new and exciting field, I found that each answer simply raised more questions. I wanted to know more about the connections between the hormone-producing glands and the immune system. I wanted to know why they were linked, and what was controlling them.

My next experiment was based on a real hunch. These days a hunch will not get you funding for your research project; you need to submit reams of paper documenting your thesis, explaining why and how your experiment will work. Intuition won't do it. Call me simpleminded, but it strikes me that if a scientist knows enough to do all this documentation ahead of time, it may not be necessary to do the experiment. Fortunately, by virtue of my position at the Institute of Medical Research in Davos, Switzerland, at that time, I had a certain amount of independence, and was able to pursue my hunches.

Enough politics. Let's get to the merits. My next experiment involved athymic nude mice, a particular genetic strain of mice that provides a wonderful "laboratory" for an immunologist. As their name suggests, these mice are born without a thymus and without hair. The gene for this breed of mouse is recessive; out of a litter of ten mice about four will be born athymic.

Athymic nude mice share the same fate as newborn mice who have had their thymuses removed. They fail to develop properly, have severe immunological problems, and die early of the same kind of wasting disease that so resembles senescence, or aging. Now, there was something about the athymic nude mice—the mice born without a thymus gland—that puzzled me. I was struck by the fact that no matter what I did, I could not get their hair to grow. When I transplanted a thymus into these mice, I was able to restore their immunity and normalize their growth, but, still, I could produce no hair. Hair growth is controlled by hormones, and it occurred to me that there might be some unknown hormone present in the brain of normal mice that was absent in these athymic mice. Why the brain? Remember, the pituitary gland is located in the brain, and so is the hypothalamus, which helps regulate the pituitary gland. Since I didn't know precisely what hormone I was looking for, I concocted a crude brain extract from the normal mice and simply injected it into the athymic mice. I never managed to get them to grow hair, but some of the mice responded very well in other ways to the brain extract. Although they remained hairless, their immune systems showed marked improvement. However, some of the mice barely showed any improvement, and I couldn't figure out why. It was utterly mysterious.

I studied my notes and scrutinized my lab techniques looking for some explanation as to why the experiment would have produced such inconsistent results; reactions that were as different as night and day. Then it struck me. The mice who fared better had been given their injections of brain extract in the late afternoon; the mice who did not do as well were injected during the morning. Why? I began to think about circadian rhythms, the daily and seasonal hormonal fluctuations that regulate the natural life cycles of animals and humans. My laboratory provided a perfect setting to ponder such thoughts. Tucked away in the Swiss Alps, with a spectacular view of the countryside, I believe that I was as close to nature as one could be while still having the benefits of a high-tech facility. In this environment, we felt the seasonal changes acutely, and I noticed that the animals in and outside of the laboratory were also deeply affected. Back in 400 B.C., Hippocrates, the "father of modern medicine," and whose oath we still take upon becoming physicians, believed that students of medicine should first learn about the seasonal changes, and how they affect men and animals. According to Hippocrates, the seasonal cycles have a profound impact on both health and behavior, and if a physician does not understand these cycles, he cannot possibly understand what is happening to his patients. What Hippocrates knew intuitively, science has proven conclusively. Science has come up with some highly sophisticated blood tests that show that the levels of various hormones actually fluctuate from season to season throughout the year and even from hour to hour throughout the day. The changes profoundly affect the life cycles of animals and humans. I began to wonder whether changes in daily hormone production could possibly be affecting immune function. Could that explain why the mice injected at night were doing so much better than the mice injected during the morning? Since I knew that the immune system was linked to the glands that controlled growth and reproduction, I couldn't help but wonder if these daily rhythms played a role in these activities as well.

All The Difference Between Night and Day:
I Began to Think in Terms of the Pineal Gland

I began to study as much as I could about circadian daily rhythms, combing the scientific journals for articles on the pineal gland. I was studying the pineal gland because scientists had earlier established that this little gland, located deep within the brain, is the mechanism that controls circadian rhythms—including sleep/wake cycles and seasonal adjustments—in humans and animals. It had also been earlier established that the pineal gland exerts this control through the production of a hormone called melatonin. In my quest for more information, I joined the newly formed European Pineal Study Group and attended a scientific conference on the pineal in Jerusalem. Notably, I found myself the sole immunologist in attendance, adrift in a sea of pineal experts.

I realized that pineal research, long neglected, was attracting the attention of more and more scientists. Their work helped me to focus my research. I found some of what they were doing to be quite fascinating. For example, one study showed that melatonin levels dropped significantly as animals aged. Yet another study that I found to be particularly intriguing reported that blind people with a rare condition called retrolental fibrosis—it causes them to have absolutely no perception of light—lived significantly longer than blind people who have some light sensitivity. To me, this strongly suggested that reactions to light and dark, and shifts in light and dark cycles might somehow affect longevity. From this I theorized that sleep/wake cycles may also play a role. If this was true, disrupting natural light cycles might alter life span.

This much I knew: Light is very important for the regulation of circadian cycles and pineal function. The pineal gland detects the presence of light and will react either by producing more or less melatonin. I devised an experiment to determine the effect of constant light on the growth and development of mice.

I isolated a group of male and female mice and raised them under permanent artificial light. For the first few generations, the mice developed normally, mated, had litters, and lived out their typical life span. By the fourth generation, however, the difference in the mice was striking. The mice no longer looked like healthy mice: Their muscles began to shrink, they grew wrinkled, they developed bald patches on their fur, their thymus glands (where the T cells are stored) developed fatty tissue, and their immune response was poor. They looked like tired, little old mice. They rapidly aged and died young. By keeping the mice under permanent light, and by preventing them from experiencing the normal day/night and sleep/wake cycle, I had actually produced precocious aging.

Why did it take four generations of mice for this to happen? I think that it is because circadian cycles are so imprinted in our nature—are so basic to life itself—that it takes several generations to erase this biological mandate. These cycles are passed from parent to child, and the memory of these cycles continues long after the cycle is disrupted. But when an animal loses its cyclicity, its ability to adapt to the daily rhythms of life, it will quickly age and die before its time. As I would soon discover, the same is true for humans.

As a result of these experiments, I changed the entire focus of my research. I felt compelled to learn more about the pineal gland, the master of circadian cycles, and the fascinating hormone that the pineal produces, melatonin. I was struck by a thought that, at the time, seemed utterly fantastic: Could the pineal be the master of our destiny? Had I finally found the orchestra leader?

CHAPTER 3
Finding the Aging Clock

"Always doubt what you believe."

—EPICTETUS

My research had persuaded me that my preconceptions about aging were wrong. I could no longer accept the conventional wisdom that aging occurred as individual cells gave out, one after another, at random. On the contrary, everything that I had learned about the interrelationship of our bodily systems and the glands and organs that comprise them had convinced me that nature had put so much care into the design of our bodies that the notion that aging had been left to chance was inconceivable. I knew that somewhere in our brain there had to be an aging clock, a chief regulator that controlled the aging process. From infancy, through puberty, through our reproductive years and beyond, we follow a preordained schedule of events that are well timed and so highly orchestrated that somewhere there had to be a "conductor." I also had an intuitive feeling that I had already identified the clock, but that I did not know it, that somewhere in the tens of thousands of pages of notes that I had taken in the course of performing hundreds of experiments, the aging clock had already revealed itself. However, like so many scientists who become fixated on one piece of the puzzle, I had become too nearsighted to see the truth. I was either in the midst of an experiment, or planning my next one, or too busy to step back and get the perspective I needed to find the missing piece of the puzzle. Sensing this, I knew that I needed time for reflection.

I have always believed that to be a true scientist, one must be more than a skilled technician. Although it is important to know how to devise the right experiments, how to execute them with precision, and how to properly record and interpret data, a scientist who is proficient only in these skills accomplishes only half the job. In reality, a true scientist must also be something of a philosopher. In other words, I think that gathering and interpreting results is not enough. After an experiment is completed and results are obtained, a scientist needs to pause and think and reflect on what we might call the big picture. It is important to look up from our own work and to see how it fits into a broader context. This is the process of synthesizing, or of combining findings with other findings to develop a coherent theory or explanation of why things are the way they are.

I have often thought that my most important breakthroughs resulted not from work done in the laboratory—although I am very proud of my laboratory research—but from the quiet hours I spent reflecting on my results and their wider implications. It was during these thoughtful periods of synthesis that I was able, as you might say, to see the forest through the trees, and that I began to develop the theory—or, if you will, philosophy—that finally led me to identify the aging clock.

In the previous chapter, I described my research on the endocrine system, the hormone-producing system of glands that regulates the most important aspects of our lives, including how we grow and develop physically and sexually. I also described my research on the immune system, whose special cells protect us against disease. I explained how I had devoted years of research to demonstrating that there was a connection between these two systems, and how eventually I did establish that the two systems are intertwined, and that the hormones of the endocrine system are in constant communication with the special cells of the immune system.

When I finally had the time for reflection, I was struck by the fact that the immune system and the endocrine system are so closely linked. I spent a great deal of time pondering why these two systems should be so closely connected. I knew that it wasn't just by chance. The human body is an exquisitely designed machine and nature has taken great pains to fine-tune and perfect all our vital parts. If nature had linked the endocrine system to the immune system, and moreover made it such a critical, important link, there had to be a compelling reason. At this point the philosopher in me took over, and the more I pondered this synergistic relationship, the more I realized that the connections between these two systems were more profound than I had first imagined.

To understand what I mean, you, too, need to step back and view the big picture, and consider the niche that we occupy in our world. We are but one species on an earth filled with literally over one million species. What makes us (and each other animal species) different is our unique genetic identity. A complex mix of genetic material is what gives us our specific identities. For example, human DNA does not look exactly like monkey DNA and neither of these look exactly like dog DNA. Each species has its own particular genetic code. Even within the same species, there are subtle differences that can distinguish one animal, or one person, from another. Your DNA does not look exactly like your neighbor's or, for that matter, your sibling's. That is why DNA testing has become such an important tool in identifying criminals.

Sometimes, because we humans are the dominant species, we forget that we are part of an ecosystem, and that life for many species in our ecosystem can be hazardous. The fundamental reason a species becomes extinct is because for some reason—starvation, disease, chemical contamination—it becomes unable to mate or reproduce. For example, peregrine falcons were threatened with extinction because pesticides entering their food chain altered their DNA, causing their egg shells to become too soft. Obviously, when a species cannot reproduce, it cannot pass on its unique genetic identity to future generations. The line cannot continue. Absent reproduction, there can be no continuation of a species, man or beast. Absent sexual attraction and sex (or a test tube substitute for it), there would be no possibility of reproduction.

All right then. We know that what makes us unique, both as a species and as individuals, is the genetic material that we carry at a cellular level. We know that if our line is to continue, we must be able to reproduce and pass this genetic material on. In order to reproduce, we need to keep our bodies healthy and strong, and our genetic material safe and intact. Viewed in this larger context, it becomes apparent that the job of our immune system is not just to *protect us* from disease, but to *protect our species* from extinction. By protecting us and our cells, our immune system permits us to reproduce and transmit our identity as a species and as individuals into future generations.

The immune system protects us from invading bacteria and viruses that can cause infection. The immune system is also an internal surveillance system that continuously monitors our bodies in order to detect and neutralize abnormal cells that can destroy DNA. One of the major jobs of the immune system is to distinguish our own cells from foreign cells, to differentiate between what immunologists call "self" and "nonself." It knows what cells belong in our bodies, and what cells do not, and when it identifies the latter, it attacks them. Without our immune systems, we would either be too weak to reproduce or, if we did reproduce, we would transmit defective genetic material. In either case, our species would eventually become extinct. The immune system, therefore, is the guardian of our genetic legacy.

Clearly then, nature knew what it was doing when it linked the immune system with the endocrine system, which controls reproduction. In the process of protecting us and keeping us well, the immune system makes it possible for the act of reproduction to occur, and without it, we would lose our identity as a species. We would lose our ability to pass our DNA on to future generations, and we would vanish.

With this in mind, I decided that it was time to step back yet again and try to gain a still broader point of view. Here we have the immune system connected to the endocrine system, and together these systems function to help ensure our survival as individuals and as a species. How else, I wondered, are they united in this common purpose?

This question led me, of course, back to the pineal gland.

By this time, science had repeatedly shown that the pineal gland, the regulator of regulators, helps control and harmonize the functioning of our reproductive (endocrine) and immune systems. For example, science had taught us that it is instructions issued by the pineal that command animals to migrate to their breeding grounds and to mate. The pineal also controls the onset of puberty in humans. Other studies—some performed in my own laboratories—had shown that the pineal, through the release of the hormone melatonin, affects the function of our immune systems.

Why, I began to wonder, had science assigned to the pineal gland the supervision of these two systems—systems that define and determine the essence and continuation of life itself? *What else*, I began to wonder, could this remarkable gland do? Could its power extend even beyond these two systems, and if so, *how far?*

Call it deductive reasoning, call it logic, call it a pure leap of faith. I had a feeling that I was closing in on a target that had always eluded detection. Could it be, I hypothesized, that the pineal gland was the body's aging clock? Could the pineal gland be the mechanism in the body that governs and controls how we age?

I decided that to test my hypothesis—to determine whether there was any real basis for my intuition—I needed to know everything that could be known about melatonin, the hormone secreted, primarily during the night, by the pineal gland. Keep in mind that by this time pineal experts had established that melatonin production declines as we humans (and other animals) age. Of course to them, this was just another of those inevitable facts of aging. To me, when viewed in the context of the pineal's role as the regulator of the endocrine and immune systems, it was a revelation. *What they perceived to be only a symptom of aging, I began to view as the cause.*

I knew that melatonin was not like other hormones. I had seen in my own experiments the devastating effect that a disruption in melatonin production can cause. When we kept mice under continuous light, so that their melatonin production was decreased and erratic, their immune function was depressed and they aged prematurely and died young. In addition, within four generations they stopped reproducing altogether. It struck me that if I could accelerate aging by interfering with the pineal's ability to produce melatonin, then I ought to be able to slow down the aging process and restore youthful vigor. If I could take a young animal and make it old, I ought to be able to do the reverse—rejuvenate an old, tired animal. I believed that I could do this by supplementing melatonin levels later in life, at the point in time at which naturally occurring levels began to decline.

To determine whether melatonin levels were really influencing the aging process, I devised a rigorous experiment, the nature and startling results of which I will now describe.

FROM OLD TO YOUNG

In fall of 1985, I began the first of what would be many experiments testing the effect of administering melatonin supplements to older mice. To perform my first experiment, I selected healthy male mice that were nineteen months old. Since members of this particular breed of mouse live to be about twenty-four months, nineteen months is the human equivalent of about sixty-five years of age. I divided the mice into two groups. The first group of mice was given melatonin in its evening drinking water. The second group was given regular tap water. Other than the difference in evening drinking water, the mice were treated exactly the same. They ate the same diet and lived under the same conditions. In order to assure regular and uniform drinking habits, we removed the drinking bottles from both groups every morning and returned the bottles to the cages at night.

Based on earlier research (my own and that of others), I suspected that the melatonin supplements would probably have a positive effect on the immune function, and would thus keep the animals healthier longer. But I wasn't sure what other effects, if any, melatonin might have.

At first, I could detect very little difference between the two groups of mice. Within five months, however, the difference between the two groups was astonishing. The untreated mice began to display the expected signs and symptoms of old age—of senescence. They lost muscle mass, they developed bald patches, their eyes grew cloudy with cataracts, their digestion slowed down, and so, generally, did they. In sum, they seemed worn out and tired—they were winding down and becoming old.

On the other hand, the melatonin-treated mice looked, and behaved, like their grandchildren. The mice on melatonin had actually grown more fur and continued to boast thick, shiny coats. Their eyes were clear and cataract-free, their digestion had improved, and, instead of growing thin and wasted in the manner of the nonmelatonin-treated mice, they maintained their strength and muscle tone. The vigor and energy with which they moved around their cage resembled the behavior of mice half their age.

Most importantly, the melatonin-treated mice lived longer, much longer! The untreated mice, having reached their expected life span of about twenty-four months (seventy to seventy-five years in human terms), began to die. Yet the melatonin mice lived on and on—an astonishing six months longer, which in human terms would amount to gaining an extra twenty-five years of life, or living well past a hundred.

Moreover, the mice lived their added years in strong, healthy bodies. Later, when I examined the mice to determine their cause of death, I found that most of untreated mice had died of cancer, which is common for their breed and age. However, much to my surprise, the melatonin-treated mice had remained disease-free throughout their extended lives. Their organs had shrunk, which is typical of old age, but they did not suffer or die from cancer.

I think it is fair to say that what we accomplished in this experiment was remarkable. We had succeeded in reversing the aging process in these animals, we had managed to extend their lifetimes by nearly a third, and we had kept them vital and healthy until they died at a ripe old age. Those results aside, what this experiment revealed about aging was even more remarkable. This experiment proved that disease is not an inevitable part of aging, and that it is possible for us not only to live longer lives, but to live them in strong, disease-free, healthy bodies. Senescence, the downward spiral that we have come to associate with aging, does not have to occur. Melatonin can stop the spiral.

We didn't rely solely on our eyes or the passage of time to document the startling and dramatic rejuvenating effects of melatonin. We performed a battery of tests to gather more objective, unbiased data. We knew that the melatonin-treated animals certainly looked to the naked eye to be substantially healthier and more vigorous, but we wanted more concrete evidence of their rejuvenation. We therefore looked at the state of their immune system, because, as we have seen, when an animal ages, its immune function declines. If the melatonin supplements had restored immune function to youthful levels, this would demonstrate not simply a rejuvenated appearance, but a true physiological rejuvenation. Here is how we conducted the test: There is a chemical that when applied to the skin of younger mice causes inflammation, but when applied to the skin of older mice provokes no such response. The reason that older mice do not react to the chemical is that older mice have a weakened immune response. We rubbed this chemical on the skin of mice from both groups. The mice that had not received melatonin responded to the chemical in exactly the same way that older mice consistently do. They did not show any signs of inflammation. In other words, the reaction was what could be expected from mice of their advanced age. The melatonin-treated mice, however, showed a rapid and strong immune response, similar to that exhibited by much younger animals. This demonstrated that the immune response of the melatonin-treated mice had been restored to more youthful levels. But we wanted still more confirmation.

We also checked for thyroid function, because it, too, tends to show signs of decline in older animals. The thyroid gland secretes hormones that regulate metabolism by increasing the oxygen consumption of cells. In young animals, thyroid hormone levels drop at night, indicating a slowing down of their metabolism, which is appropriate at times of rest. However, in older animals, thyroid hormone levels remain high at night. In the mice that did not receive melatonin, thyroid function remained high at night as would be expected in mice of their age. In the melatonin-treated mice, however, the thyroid hormone levels fell at night, just as they do in younger animals. Clearly, melatonin supplementation had corrected many of the so-called normal symptoms of aging.

But the best news is yet to come.

As scientific protocol demands, we repeated this experiment several times to make sure that we could duplicate the results, so that our remarkable work wouldn't be dismissed as a fluke or aberration. Each subsequent time, the older animals treated with melatonin showed dramatically improved health, and lived much longer than normal. But in one of our experiments, in which we used male and female mice, we discovered something new and exciting. Both the males and females displayed the sexual prowess of much younger mice. In fact, right up until their death, these mice were sexually active. This would be the equivalent of one-hundred-year-old men and women showing the sexual interest and stamina of people a third their age!

Consistent with this was our finding that there was a noticeable improvement in the size and condition of the sex organs of the melatonin-treated mice as opposed to the untreated mice. In female mice, the ovaries (where sex hormones are produced) typically shrivel up with age, as they do in human females after menopause. However, in the melatonin-treated animals the ovaries remained their youthful size. In fact, at twenty-four months, which is the human equivalent of about seventy-five, the weight of the ovaries of the mice on melatonin was double that of the untreated mice. This was comparable to the ovarian size of mice half their age, and suggests that these mice have retained some of their youthful sexual function.

In male mice, the results were no less dramatic. The testes of mice (where sperm and testosterone are produced) also shrink as mice age. However, the testes of the melatonin-treated mice showed no signs of shrinkage and, in fact, were comparable to the testes of much younger animals.

It is our belief that there is a direct connection between the youthful state of the sex organs and the level of sexual activity. Based on these findings, we have no doubt that melatonin can permanently delay the aging of sexual and reproductive function. It is a true sex-enhancing hormone.

For me, these were the most exciting discoveries of all, not just because they showed that melatonin helped to reinvigorate the sex lives of older animals (and the implications for humans are obvious), not just because they further reinforced our belief that the systems that control our development, immune function, and reproduction are linked, *but because they showed that in addition to being able to extend life, we were able to extend a life in a way that made it worth living*. This to me is the driving force behind our research. After all, if the years we add cannot be joyous ones, then what purpose would be served by adding them? But here was concrete evidence that it was possible to live more than a century, and still be sexy, vital, lusty, and youthful in all the best senses of those words.

These experiments forever changed my vision of aging. I was now tantalized by the concept that we could exercise much more control over the aging process than we had ever imagined, but I also knew that we needed to learn how to exercise this control. I had taken the first important step. I had managed to reverse aging. I had proven that through melatonin supplementation it is possible to postpone the aging process, to keep our bodies youthful and strong, to remain sexy and vital throughout our entire lives. But I also knew that what we had seen was only part of a larger story. Once again, I took a step back in order to assess our findings. Here is what we knew:

1. The pineal gland produces melatonin, primarily at night.
2. The pineal gland produces less and less melatonin as we age.

3. If melatonin supplements are taken at the time of life when melatonin levels naturally decline, the effects of aging can be reversed.

But what we did not know was why. The effect of melatonin was clear, but why and how melatonin had this age-reversing effect was still a mystery. I had a strong feeling that melatonin was not merely being produced by the pineal, but that it was actually operating on and through the pineal. In other words, I suspected that it was not solely melatonin, but the pineal gland that produces the melatonin, that controls how we age. The question was, how to determine whether this theory was true?

PROOF POSITIVE

For some time, I had been contemplating doing an experiment that to my knowledge had never been attempted before: transplanting a pineal gland from a young mouse into an old mouse. I reasoned that if a young pineal could rejuvenate an old mouse—just as the melatonin supplement rejuvenated old mice when it was placed in their night drinking water—then we would have discovered something extraordinary: that the pineal gland controlled aging.

Transplanting a pineal gland is not easy. The pineal gland of a human is about the size of a small pea; the pineal gland of a mouse is about the size of the period at the end of this sentence. It is tiny and fragile, and transplanting it from one mouse to another requires a great deal of patience and precision.

Then there was the question of where to put the transplanted pineal. Ideally, when one transplants an organ, one takes out the old organ and replaces it with the new one. This is not easy to do with a gland the size of the pineal, located in an organ as sensitive as the brain. Also, at the time I was doing the initial experiments, microsurgery technology in my laboratory was not as advanced as it is today. Thus, I knew that I would have to leave the old pineal in place. For a while, I had also considered putting the new pineal into the kidney capsule, which was often used as a transplant site in animal experiments. I debated this problem with Bill Regelson, who happened to be visiting my lab in Switzerland at the time. I consider Bill to be one of the most creative, innovative researchers in the field of aging today, and I asked him to collaborate with me on this experiment. Bill and I decided that we should transplant the pineal into the thymus, a small gland located in the sternum or back of the breastbone. As you may recall from the previous chapter, much of my earlier work had been done on the thymus, which is critical for immune function in younger animals. The thymus and the pineal have something very important in common: They are connected to the same nerve center in the brain, the superior cervical sympathetic ganglion, which runs from the base of the brain, where the pineal is located, all the way to the sternum and the thymus. Since the thymus and pineal are both fed by the same nerves, we believed that the thymus was a more natural location for the pineal than the kidney.

In our experiment, we removed young pineals from mice who were three to four months old (or the human equivalent of a teenager) and transplanted them into six twenty-month-old male mice (about age sixty-five to seventy in human years). We also transplanted pineals from young mice into female mice, aged sixteen, nineteen, and twenty-two months old (or fifty, sixty-five, and seventy in human years). To avoid rejection of the new pineal, we used special inbred mice that were the genetic equivalent of identical twins. The donor tissue was so similar to the recipient's tissue that it was readily accepted. Each procedure was performed with painstaking care under a surgical microscope. A single pineal gland in its membrane was positioned on the tip of a needle and gently inserted into the thymus of the older mice.

The mice that had received the pineal transplants, like the melatonin-treated mice in the prior experiment, appeared to grow young before our eyes. Their fur improved, their activity level increased and they looked and acted like much younger mice. Both their immune response and thyroid function were equal to those of much younger animals. The thymus glands of the transplanted mice, which are usually shrunken and atrophied in mice of their age, had been restored to their youthful size and condition. This suggested that the way melatonin restores immune function is by rejuvenating the thymus gland.

The mice that received the young pineals lived on average three months longer than normal (about ten to fifteen human years). We also saw that the younger the mice were when they received the new pineals, the longer their life span was extended. In other tests, we also saw that mice who received young pineals at age twenty-two months lived three to four months longer, approximately 20 percent longer than normal life span. Mice who received young pineals at age nineteen months lived five to six months longer, approximately 30 to 35 percent longer than normal life span. Thus, from this experiment we also learned that rejuvenation cannot be achieved if intervention comes too late. We concluded that there is a point when the body organs have become so deteriorated that rejuvenation is just not possible, and that if we are to successfully intervene and stop the aging process, intervention has to occur before the point of no return.

This experiment also raised a particularly perplexing question. You will recall that the mice that received melatonin in their drinking water lived an average six months (twenty-five human years) longer than their life expectancy. The mice that received the pineal transplants lived only an average of three months (about ten to fifteen human years) longer than expected. Why this difference? Why didn't the mice with the pineal transplants live as long as the mice receiving melatonin in their evening drinking water? If the pineal gland is the regulator of the regulators, and if it operates through its hormone melatonin, why should melatonin supplementation have a more positive effect on aging than implantation of a young pineal? As we reviewed our results and our procedures and pondered everything we knew about the regulatory role of the pineal, it occurred to us that these problematic results might be related to the fact that our subject mice had not one, but two, pineal glands. You will recall that although we had implanted new pineals into the older mice, we did not remove their old pineals. We theorized that the old pineal gland must have been telling the body to age, while the new pineal gland was in effect telling it not to age. The result was that aging was slowed down, but not to the extent that it was in the mice with a single pineal that received melatonin supplements. To return to our orchestra metaphor, it was as if the musicians were receiving conflicting directions from two different conductors.

The results of our transplantation experiments made us more curious than ever about the pineal, and heightened our conviction that it is not only instrumental in the aging process, but is, indeed, the aging clock. We had seen signs of rejuvenation in the animals that had received the pineal transplants, and we had also seen a modest increase in life span. However, we both felt that we needed more information and validation. Science is very demanding, and there were many questions still to be answered before we could say conclusively that the pineal and the pineal alone controlled aging.*

THE FINAL WORD: CROSS TRANSPLANTATION

My work next took me to Russia, where I had an opportunity to meet Vladimir Lesnikov, a young researcher whose work so impressed me that I eventually arranged for him to come work with me in Switzerland.

Lesnikov had devised a special piece of equipment

---

* One of these questions was posed by my friend and colleague the late Branislav D. Jankovic, whose work on the thymus was instrumental in forming my own theories. Jankovic suggested that we had to rule out the possibility that the rejuvenation had been triggered not by the new pineals, but by the surgery itself, which might somehow have stimulated the regeneration of the thymus, which in turn was responsible for the mice's extended life span and more youthful state. Heeding Jankovic's cautionary words, I devised yet another experiment, which if successful would verify our earlier findings. In this experiment, I transplanted not the pineal gland, but a piece of cerebral cortex tissue from young mice donors into the thymus glands of older mice. This experiment was carried out precisely the same way, and with the same painstaking detail, as the pineal transplantations. I myself was curious about what, if anything, would happen. I waited patiently and watched the mice for several months for any signs of change. No signs of rejuvenation appeared. The mice with the cerebral cortex transplants lived out their normal life spans, in their aging bodies. They grew weak, and old, and died, just like normal mice their age. This provided the necessary proof that it was not some inadvertent effect of the surgical process, but rather the pineal transplant itself that was the proximate cause of the rejuvenation.

that made it possible to perform the most intricate brain surgery on the tiniest of animal subjects. His invention, called a stereotaxic instrument, provided a three-dimensional view of the head, while allowing a surgeon to position it in precisely the right position for incredibly delicate maneuvers. Thanks to Lesnikov's ingenious invention—and his "magic hands"—we would now be able to perform the one experiment that I believed would prove without a doubt that the pineal was the true aging clock. It would, as no other experiment had yet done, reveal the power of the pineal.

The experiment we had devised was simple in concept, but excruciatingly difficult to execute. We wanted to see what would happen if we transplanted a pineal gland from a young mouse into an old mouse, and a pineal gland from an old mouse into a young mouse. By doing such a cross transplantation of pineal glands, we could see what effect, if any, the old pineal would have in a young animal, and a young pineal would have in an old animal.

This procedure was far more sophisticated than my initial pineal transplantations into the thymus. For one thing, by exchanging an old pineal for a young one, we could actually see the effect of the new pineal without it being hampered by conflicting instructions from the old pineal. If the procedure worked, the pineal could perhaps regenerate its nerve supply and be reconstituted as a normal, working gland in its correct anatomical location. This would provide a more realistic view of how the pineal functions than was obtainable by placing the transplanted pineal in the thymus. Also, we would be able to see how an old pineal would behave in a young body. I found this prospect to be particularly intriguing. I knew from past experiments that the aging clock could be slowed down, but could it also be speeded up? Would an old pineal in a young body also accelerate the aging process?

The Melatonin Miracle

This experiment posed a real challenge to even the most skilled of surgeons. Although its power and influence is enormous, the pineal is in fact extremely small. As I pointed out earlier in this chapter, in humans the pineal is about the size of a pea. In mice it is dot-sized and barely visible to the unaided eye. We could perform only a very few surgeries a day, with each session requiring about three to four days of preparation and at least several hours of surgical time. Thus, it took us weeks to finish all the operations.

For our subject group, we exchanged the pineal glands of mice aged four months (the equivalent of twenty human years) with the pineal glands of mice aged eighteen months (the equivalent of about sixty human years). For our control group, we performed sham operations on groups of four-month-old mice and eighteen-month-old mice. We removed their pineals and put them right back into the same mice. From the control group, we could determine if it was the surgery, and not the transplants, that was having an effect on health and life span.

The operations went well, and within a few months we had several cages of cross-transplanted animals living side by side.

We were careful to tag each mouse, and each surgical group was placed in their own cage, so each cage consisted of two four-month-olds, and two eighteen-month-olds. Each week, we carefully examined all the mice, checking their vital signs and taking other measures of physical health.

We began the operations in spring of 1990, and after that all we could do was to wait patiently for the results. Many months passed. Then one morning I entered the lab, glanced at the cages, and was positively alarmed by what I saw. The mice in several of the cages all appeared to be the same age—I knew this was impossible. We had carefully mixed together the young mice with the old mice so that we could see more precisely any contrasts in behavior and appearance that occurred. I immediately assumed that one of the other lab technicians had accidentally mixed them up. Yet, upon closer examination—after checking all their identification tags—I realized that the mice were indeed in the right cages.

Suddenly, the full impact of what I was seeing hit me. The reason the mice all appeared to be the same age was that the experiment had actually worked! The old mice had been rejuvenated by the young pineals!

What was even more startling, however, was the fact that the young mice with the old pineals were aging rapidly, way before their time. Both groups of mice looked precisely the same age. I was so amazed by what I saw that I ran to get my camera and took pictures. To this day, I still look at those pictures and marvel at what I see; two mice, standing side by side, one fifteen months old, one thirty months old, both looking exactly the same age. In human terms that would be the equivalent of a forty-year-old standing next to a ninety-year-old—and passing as twins.

But soon after that the "age" difference between the two groups of mice dramatically emerged. The young mice implanted with the old pineals began to whither and die, about 30 percent earlier than normal. The old mice implanted with the young pineals, however, lived on average 30 percent longer, and maintained their youthful, vigorous bodies until the very end of life, which was about thirty-three months, or in human terms, around 105 years. Later examination would reveal that the thymus glands of the old mice who had received the young pineals had regenerated, whereas the thymus glands of the young mice who had received the old pineals had withered.

What happened to the control mice who underwent the sham operations? Nothing. They lived out their lives quite normally, showing no signs of anything out of the ordinary.

From this experiment, I concluded that I had found the true aging clock and finally understood not only *how* we age, but *why* we age. As I had suspected, the pineal is the key. A young pineal sends a youthful message throughout the body, keeping the body healthy and strong. Once the pineal ages, however, it sends quite a different message, telling the body that we are old and that it is time to wind down. One by one, the various systems follow the pineal's lead, until we grow old and die.

As you may remember, when I administered melatonin to the older mice in one of my earlier experiments, I was able to significantly extend their life and rejuvenate their bodies. I believe that melatonin supplementation helped bring the pineal back to its youthful state, and in so doing altered the message it was sending to the rest of the body and restored normal cyclicity or balance to the body. From these experiments I concluded that maintaining melatonin at youthful levels in older humans would have the same positive effects.

So the pineal is the aging clock. In the next chapter we will take a closer look at the pineal gland to understand its powers, what it does, and how precisely it functions in our bodies as the clock of aging.

CHAPTER 4

The Pineal Gland: Your "Third Eye"

The pineal gland is the body's aging clock, the internal timer that controls the aging process. It releases the hormone melatonin, which transmits instructions to other body systems that tells them how and when to age. We age because our pineal glands tell us to. With the benefit of hindsight, this is not surprising, since nearly all of our vital bodily functions are somehow under the control of the pineal gland. The pineal gland is the regulator of the endocrine system, the hormones that control all human activities, including when we sleep, how we grow, and even our sexual development. Clearly, the pineal gland has a profound effect on every aspect of our lives, and has probably performed these functions since the beginning of our time on earth. In many ways, we owe our very survival to this tiny, hardworking gland.

In mammals, including humans, the pineal is set deep within the center of the brain and does not have direct access to light. Instead, it "sees" through our eyes. Light passes through the pupil and is focused on the retina, the light-sensitive layer that lines the interior of the eye. From the retina, a message is relayed through the optic nerve to the middle brain and the suprachiasmatic nuclei, a cluster of nerve cells in the hypothalamus. The hypothalamus is a center within the middle brain that also serves as a sort of internal clock for the body. Each day, the light that is "let in" by the eyes sets the timing mechanism on the suprachiasmatic nucleus. Each night, the suprachiasmatic nucleus sends a signal along a pathway down into the spinal cord, back up through the neck, and into the pineal gland. The amount of light that is registered on the pineal through the eyes determines the production of melatonin. Light suppresses melatonin production; therefore, the duration of daylight, which varies according to the season, affects the ebb and flow of melatonin.

The pineal gland enables us to live in harmony with our environment. Long before there were clocks to mark the hours, calendars to count the days, or satellites spinning through space to track the weather, we humans relied on nature's cues to know when to rest, work, play, and even mate. These cues were given to us by our pineal gland and our pineal gland performs the same functions today. For example, in ancient times when the sun set, and the earth grew dark, the pineal gland produced melatonin, which made our ancestors sleepy. Today, although we have clocks to tell us the time of day and night, our bodies still follow a natural rhythm set by the pineal gland through the release of melatonin. As the seasons changed, the pineal gland, through its control of other hormones, helped our ancestors regulate their body temperature to adjust to the changing cycles in weather. This enabled our ancestors to move freely from climate to climate, in search of food, and gave them an edge over other species that could not adapt. The pineal gland even regulates the release of hormones that help new mothers forge a tight bond with their offspring. It is this bond that creates the maternal instinct that drives a mother to protect her young. This maternal instinct is as necessary for the survival of our species today as it was many thousands of years ago.

The influence of the pineal gland is no less profound in animals. In the spring, the lengthening of the days is detected by the pineal gland, which signals to migrating animals that it is time to begin their spring journey. In the fall, when the days grow shorter, the pineal gland triggers the growth of fur on animals so they can survive the winter chill, and this same gland also signals to hibernating mammals that it is time to start fattening up for the long sleep ahead. When winter ends, the pineal gland alerts hibernating animals that it is time to wake up by turning up their metabolism, and signals to nonhibernating animals that it is time to shed their heavy winter coats for lighter, spring coats.

Unlike animals, who are still very much subject to the whims of nature, we humans are not. Thanks to modern conveniences like electric lights and air conditioning, we can control our external environment to some degree. Yet we still rely on the pineal gland to regulate our circadian rhythms, the daily cyclical release of hormones that governs all of our activities from eating to sleeping to metabolism. The best example of what our circadian rhythms do occurs when these rhythms are upset, as when we travel to another time zone. For days after a transatlantic or transcontinental flight, our sleeping patterns, our eating patterns, and our thought processes are disrupted. When ultimately we do adjust to a new time zone and climate, it is because the pineal gland has made the necessary adjustments. (The topic of jet lag, and how to avoid it, is covered in more detail in Chapter 13.)

We are not the first to write about the wonders of the pineal, and we doubt that we'll be the last. The pineal has been the subject of speculation, reverence, and even controversy for the past twenty-five hundred years, and it undoubtedly will continue to be through the next millennium. French philosopher René Descartes said that the soul operated through the pineal gland, an assertion that outraged the theologians of his day. Hindu mystics called the pineal the "third eye" and believed that it was the site from which the soul departed the body during the highest meditative states. It's interesting to note that these philosophers and mystics somehow sensed the importance of the pineal, even though their scientist contemporaries did not. Only within the past three decades have scientists begun to study the pineal gland seriously. Since then, we have learned some fascinating things about it.

The intuition of the Hindu mystics was very much on point. The pineal did start out as a "third eye" in lower animals. We can see the vestiges of this third eye in the Tuatura, a New Zealand lizard that actually has a small indentation on its forehead that allows light to fall directly on its pineal. Some scientists believe that at one time the pineal did indeed serve as an eye for some reptiles. Oddly enough, the pineal never developed into a real eye. Rather, nature adapted it for other even more important uses.

In many birds (who share common ancestry with reptiles), the pineal is instrumental in migration. Birds rely on a number of signposts to keep them on course as they traverse the globe, including the position of the sun and changes in the daily light/dark cycles. In birds, the pineal sits close to the skull, which is transparent, so light passes through it. Studies have shown that if the skulls of migrating sparrows are painted with black ink so that light cannot pass through, the migrating birds become hopelessly lost.

There is also evidence that birds may be able to detect variations in the earth's magnetic field, and thus have a built-in natural compass. The pineal gland may be this compass. This is not as strange as it sounds.

With its metal core, the earth is like a giant magnet spinning through space. With a mass much greater than the earth's, the sun also exerts a strong electromagnetic pull on the earth, and to a lesser degree so does the moon. As the earth orbits around the sun, and the moon orbits around the earth, the earth's electromagnetic fields vary. The pineal gland of many animals, including humans, is believed to be sensitive to magnetic forces. Through their pineal glands, migrating birds may sense changes in the earth's electromagnetic fields, which in turn can help them find their way. This is how birds can fly thousands of miles away from their summer homes during winter migration periods, and still return to the precise location from which they departed months earlier to nest and breed in the spring.

Studies have also shown that the human pineal gland may sense and react to other types of electromagnetic fields, such as those emitted by simple household appliances such as clocks and hair dryers. In fact, several studies have shown that exposure to electromagnetic fields can actually interfere with the evening production of melatonin. Although the theory is controversial and losing force among epidemiological authorities, some researchers believe that exposure to electromagnetic fields may be a possible cause of many different types of cancers.

The human pineal is very tiny. It is larger in children than in adults, and shrinks as we get older. For some as yet undiscovered reason, women have slightly larger pineal glands than men. Perhaps this should not surprise us, though, considering the fact that women's lives are so closely regulated by cycles—the twenty-eight-day menstrual cycle being a case in point. It's also interesting to note that women typically live longer than men, and we can speculate as to whether this, too, might be related to their larger pineal glands.

Ironically, until the past three decades scientists considered the pineal to be of minor, if any, importance. No one knew quite what to make of it. When scientists removed the pineal from animals, nothing of visible or obvious significance resulted. Consequently, they theorized that the pineal was just a vestigial organ that no longer had any function, a body part of no greater consequence (and perhaps less) than our tonsils or appendix. Of course, we now know this view was incorrect. One reason that removing the pineal may have appeared to have no immediate effect is because—as we have since learned—the glands comprising the endocrine system (of which the pineal is one) are closely linked, and if one gland is removed, very often the others may compensate, at least partly, for the loss. Moreover, we now know that the impact of removing the pineal varies according to stage of development; removing a pineal during an animal's infancy has a very different effect from removing it at a later point in life.

Nearly a century ago, researchers realized that the pineal gland played a significant role in sexual development. As early as 1889, a physician described a bizarre case involving a four-year-old boy who was already showing signs of puberty. The physician also discovered that the boy had a pineal tumor. This case caused some researchers to suspect that the pineal gland secreted a substance that delayed sexual function and the onset of puberty, and that the pineal tumor might have inhibited the production of this substance.

More than a half century later, in 1958, two researchers, A. B. Lerner and J. D. Case, isolated the mysterious substance and named it melatonin, after the Greek words *melas*, meaning black, and *tosos*, meaning labor. They chose this name because, after isolating the substance, they had applied it to the skin of laboratory frogs, and, when they did this, the substance interacted with melanophores, pigment cells in the skin, and lightened or darkened the frogs' skin. Some animals, including frogs and certain reptiles such as chameleons, are able to change their skin color almost instantaneously to camouflage themselves and hide from predators, and the pineal controls this potentially life-saving function. In 1963, melatonin was recognized as a hormone, after it was shown to affect sexual function when injected into rats.

The more attention that researchers gave to this "new" hormone, the more intriguing things they discovered. They found that melatonin production was inhibited by exposure to light, and that, in fact, melatonin levels were subject to a daily cycle, rising at night and falling during the day. They noticed that blood levels of melatonin at night are ten times what they are during the day. They found that since melatonin is broken down and used within hours after it is produced, there are hardly any traces of melatonin in the blood during the day. When researchers gave people melatonin, they found that it made them sleepy, and from this scientists concluded that melatonin must play an important role in controlling the sleep/wake cycle.

Scientists learned still other curious facts about melatonin. They found that melatonin levels are higher in children than in adults, and that blood levels of melatonin fall off dramatically in old age. Indeed, we think that this decline in melatonin among the elderly is very likely why older people have so much difficulty sleeping. Scientists also discovered that cancer patients and others who are chronically ill typically had abnormally low melatonin levels. Bit by bit, scientists began to piece together the picture of the pineal gland and melatonin, and the more they learned, the bigger the picture became.

MELATONIN: THE SEX CONNECTION

In all animals, including humans, melatonin plays a major role in sexuality and reproduction, and we discuss this in greater detail in Part III. For now it is important to note that melatonin has direct control over the reproductive cycles of many animals. Unlike humans, who can conceive at any season of the year, most animals have a specific time during which they can conceive—a so-called breeding season. During this time and only during this time, do females ovulate (this is known as the estrus cycle) and males produce sperm. Such a breeding season is very important for the survival of a species because it ensures that the young will be born during the optimal conditions, usually during spring and summer, when the weather is good and food is plentiful. Sheep conceive in the fall, carry their young for six months, and give birth in the spring when the fields are green and ripe for grazing. Many birds build their nests and lay their eggs in the early spring, so that they will hatch while the weather is still warm, and so the new babies can learn to fly and hunt for food before cold weather sets in. We know that animals respond to these seasonal changes because the pineal commands them to. In animals, sexual behavior is governed by light and the corresponding fluctuations in melatonin. Changes in day length result in changes in melatonin production, which either turn on or shut down the appropriate sex hormones. There have been some fascinating animal studies that have shown that when light cycles are artificially altered, animals' reproductive cycles are altered accordingly. For example, if rodents are forced to live under conditions of shortened light cycles, mimicking the short days of winter, males experience testicular regression and females suffer an inhibition of the estrus cycle. On the other hand, when the light cycles are adjusted to mimic the long days of spring and summer, the rats become fecund.

Hibernation, as we mentioned earlier, is another activity critical to survival that is regulated by the pineal. During animal hibernation, the systems of the body wind down, much as they do during human sleep. The body temperature drops, the heart rate slows, the cells produce less energy, and the animal goes into a deep, sound slumber. Many animals mate before they hibernate, so that their young will be born in the spring. In order to survive the long months in hibernation, animals need sufficient fat stores so that they don't starve, and so that their bodies have energy to keep going. During hibernation, melatonin regulates how and when the stored fat is consumed. Shortly before it is time for an animal to wake from its long winter's sleep, the animal begins to burn fat at a more rapid pace. In fact, the more rapid consumption of fat stores is itself a signal to the animal that it is time to awaken. Like clockwork, when the snow melts, the flowers bloom, and migrating animals return, hibernating animals are ready to rejoin the world.

Even though human beings do not have a breeding season, there is evidence that our ancestors most certainly did. A comprehensive study reported in *The Journal of Reproductive Rhythms* investigated whether there was a seasonal pattern in human births. Researchers reviewed millions of birth records in Northern Hemisphere countries, all of which were in the temperate zone and had more or less the same seasonal cycles. Although the researchers took pains to point out that humans are fertile and give birth all year round, they did find two notable annual peaks in births—one in late December and early January, and the other in midsummer. The study noted that the timing of the births meant that the conceptions occurred either in early spring or early fall, when the temperature is normally between fifty and seventy degrees. For some reason, these weather conditions appear to promote fertility in both men and women. No one could explain why these conditions would stimulate fertility, but there is speculation that this may be a vestige of an ancient and long forgotten human breeding season.

Gone are the days when human beings lived in sync with their environment. We no longer live by nature's rules: A flick of a switch floods nature's dark nights with artificial light. Our homes and workplaces are climate-controlled. We are protected from the cold of winter by central heating and from the heat of summer by central air conditioning. Although these modern conveniences have certainly made life a lot more comfortable, some scientists believe that the rise in infertility in Western nations could be due to the fact that we live in what are, in effect, artificial surroundings, far removed from nature's cues, and, perhaps, from our natural breeding season as well.

As we have said, in many animals, melatonin secretion varies according to length of season and day. Human studies show that for men this is no longer the case. Their melatonin levels are constant year-round. However, women are different. Their melatonin levels are still subject to seasonal cyclicity. A recent study shows that women produce less melatonin in the summer when the days are long, and more melatonin in the winter when the days are short. Notably, researchers have found that men are more likely to suffer a disruption of their natural cycles when exposed to artificial light than are women. The researchers were unable to explain gender differences in melatonin production, but once again we suggest that the larger size of the female pineal gland may play a protective role in helping women stay attuned to their natural rhythms.

Melatonin Through the Ages

Although we human beings like to believe that we are the masters of our fate, and that we are calling the shots, cyclicity is deeply ingrained in us and it affects many of our daily activities. With rare exceptions, human beings tend to follow the same cues for wake and sleep. Sitting in a dark room tends to make most of us feel groggy and relaxed, while sitting in a brightly lit room tends to make us feel wide awake and alert. We tend to feel hunger at roughly the same times, and most of us eat three meals a day, with more or less the same time intervals between meals. Before we even leave the womb, many of our daily rhythms are already established. Not only are animals born in sync with the climate in which they live, they are born knowing precisely the right time to hibernate, migrate, or mate. This knowledge is passed from mother to fetus during pregnancy, and from mother to child during breast-feeding via melatonin. In humans, melatonin passes through the placenta from the mother to the fetus, and is also present in breast milk, which contains high levels of melatonin at night and undetectable levels during the day. Newborn infants do not begin cycling their own melatonin until they are several days old. The melatonin cycles in the mother's breast milk help to reinforce normal day/night cycles, and may even help to synchronize the infant's sleep patterns with those of his parents. As early as the first few days of life, babies begin cycling their own supplies of melatonin, but the rhythm is not fully established until the first year of life. Perhaps this explains why some babies are such erratic sleepers. We have wondered whether some of the crankiness and restlessness sometimes associated with bottle-fed babies is the result of their failure to receive the mother's dose of melatonin that is passed in breast milk, rather than the result of the colic on which it is usually blamed.

The nursing mother's supplies of melatonin help her produce prolactin, the hormone that encourages milk production, and this itself has other interesting effects. Prolactin helps maintain animals in a calm, restful state and also plays a role governing bonding and defense of the young. Levels of prolactin are particularly high in birds while they are brooding their eggs. When prolactin is administered to humans, it generates feelings of peace and serenity, and even affection. At the same time that a new mother is pumping prolactin, she is bonding with her newborn, experiencing the first sensations of maternal love.

Melatonin levels continue to rise in children until about age seven. During the first few years of life, most children tend to nap at roughly the same time during the day. Up until about the second or third year, children usually nap twice a day—once in the midmorning, and once in the early afternoon. At about age three, children begin to nap just once a day, in the afternoon, and by age four or five they tend to stop napping altogether. Although this pattern has not yet been adequately studied, we suspect that fluctuations in melatonin levels must somehow promote the napping cycle, and for good reason. During sleep, the pituitary gland produces growth hormone, which as its name suggests, stimulates growth. In children, the greatest growth spurt coincides with the periods when they sleep the most, from infancy through age three.

When children reach adolescence and their bodies grow, so does their blood volume. As a result, blood levels of melatonin become more dilute. This reduction in melatonin levels signals the body that it is time for the onset of puberty. Once the melatonin levels drop, it is a signal for the body to pump higher levels of two sex hormones, LH (luteinizing hormone) and

FSH (follicle-stimulating hormone). The change in the hormonal environment leads to the menstrual cycle in girls, and sperm production in boys.

Starting at about age forty-five, melatonin levels begin their steepest decline. We lose the ability to properly cycle melatonin, and the "aging process" begins. Women enter menopause, and although men remain fertile, they begin to show signs of diminishing sexual function. These, and all other signs of aging, are a direct result of the breakdown of the pineal and the loss of the body's natural cycles. What is actually happening is that the pineal is losing its hold over the rest of the body, or in other words, the conductor is running out of steam.

THE REGULATOR OF THE REGULATORS

The pineal gland is regarded as the "regulator" of the regulators because it rules the endocrine system, which in turn produces the hormones that control so many of our bodily functions. Through its hold over the endocrine system, the pineal controls the activities of virtually every cell in the body, affecting such diverse functions as reproduction, body temperature, kidney function, immunity, sleep, and growth and development. All of this, in addition to regulating the aging process, is under the province of the single pineal gland. How does this tiny gland perform so many vital roles? It is a "smart" gland that does just the right thing at the right time with both speed and precision.

The pineal uses melatonin to maintain the body's balance or equilibrium. Melatonin is what is called a state-dependent hormone. Unlike estrogen, which has a direct effect on specific organs such as the ovaries, or testosterone, which has a direct effect on the testes, melatonin operates indirectly to affect all organs. Its job is to regulate the levels of other hormones, and to maintain the balance, or homeostasis, of the body and thereby help the other hormones do their job. When melatonin levels rise, this inhibits the production of certain hormones; when melatonin levels drop, this stimulates the production of other hormones. Melatonin fine-tunes the production of hormones so that the body doesn't produce levels that are too high or too low.

The pineal continuously monitors the body to see what needs to be done, where it needs to be done, and the best way to do it. Although the pineal is not literally a "third eye" in the optical sense, in a way that's precisely the role it plays in our bodies. The pineal "watches over" our internal environment, and at the same time helps us adjust to our external environment. From deep within the brain, the pineal serves as a central switchboard, integrating messages transmitted to and from other points in the brain, and helping each of our glands respond to these messages.

Our bodies are constantly being bombarded with various stresses and stimuli that require instant adjustments. Although we are not even conscious of any of these stressors, our bodies detect them immediately, and respond to them automatically. For example, when we walk into a cold room, our body temperature goes down and we need to warm ourselves up. Or, if we are exposed to a virus, we need to quickly produce the right antibody to deactivate it before it can do us harm. In order to respond to these stressors, the body needs energy. Every cell in the body requires the right amount of energy at the right time to do its job. Every conceivable human activity—whether it's blinking an eye, talking, running a marathon, or even just thinking—demands energy, or the fuel to keep the cells working. It is our belief that the pineal's primary role is to control the production and use of energy throughout the body. Through the release of melatonin and perhaps other compounds, the pineal directs energy production so that it goes where it is needed at precisely the right time, whether it is needed to repair or respond to injury, or make hormones, enzymes, or antibodies. In sum, melatonin directs the cells in the body to do whatever it takes to keep the body running like the highly efficient machine it is.

Energy production is an extremely complex biochemical process, in which the pineal plays a pivotal role. Here is a very simplified explanation of how it works. In addition to melatonin, there are many other compounds in the pineal, including TRH, thyrotropin-releasing hormone, which is also found elsewhere throughout the body. When the body needs energy, the pineal tells TRH to stimulate the pituitary gland to produce TSH, thyroid-stimulating hormone. TSH acts on the thyroid gland, a butterfly-shaped gland that lies just below the larynx. The thyroid secretes three hormones, calcitonin, triiodothyronine (T_3) and thyroxine (T_4). Calcitonin is essential for the maintenance of calcium. T_3 and T_4 are critical for the functioning of other glands and organs. They control metabolism by increasing oxygen consumption of cells to make more energy. Of the two, T_3 is the "hotter" hormone because it provides more energy to the cells. Melatonin is instrumental in the breakdown of T_4 into T_3. As more energy is required, melatonin breaks down more T_4 into T_3, creating more heat and energy.

We've told you a lot about how the pineal gland exerts its control over so many functions in the body, and to underscore the importance of the pineal gland we want to show how just one of its functions is so critical to sustaining life. Maintaining normal body temperature is fundamental to our survival and is controlled by the pineal through its modulation of thyroid

77

hormone. Warm-blooded mammals are able to regulate body temperature and to keep it within a normal range regardless of climate. That's why we humans can survive as well in Hawaii as we can in Iceland, whereas many species of birds must migrate when the weather turns cold to a more moderate climate. Unlike these birds, we have internal controls that either turn up or turn down our body temperature as needed. What would happen if we lost those controls? If our body temperature was allowed to rise above the safety zone, the results would be disastrous. As our bodies heated up, we would burn up energy at too rapid a pace, and in the process produce too much heat. As our bodies attempted to cool down, we would sweat excessively and lose valuable body fluid, which would result in serious dehydration. Eventually, this unfortunate cascade of events would lead to irreparable brain damage and death. If our body temperature was allowed to drop too low, the results would be equally deadly. First, our metabolism would slow to a crawl, our major body systems would not have the energy to function, our brains would stop working, our hearts would stop beating, and we would slip into a coma and die.

Maintaining balance within our bodies becomes progressively more difficult as we age, and as the pineal wears out, even simple tasks can become a major challenge. For example, older people often have a harder time adapting to a new environment, and a common complaint among the elderly is that they are always too cold in the winter and too hot in the summer. This is due to a loss of thyroid and pineal function. Older people in general have a more difficult time adapting to any kind of environmental variation, whether it's adjusting to temperature fluctuation, recognizing smells, tasting food, responding to sexual cues, fighting off a virus, or even knowing when it's time to sleep. In a sense, growing old is the loss of the ability to adjust to one's environment, and that is because the regulator of the regulator, the pineal gland, is breaking down.

WHY AND HOW THE PINEAL BREAKS

As scientists are beginning to recognize the importance of the pineal gland, there is more and more research being devoted to how this powerful gland ages and why it eventually breaks down. So far, there are many theories, but few solid answers.

One of the things that has long puzzled scientists is the fact that, as many of us age, our pineal glands calcify. In fact, X-rays of the pineal of an older person often show that the pineal is full of calcium deposits or so-called brain sand, and many scientists have assumed that this deterioration affects pineal function. Some have even suggested that the pineal is the "stalking horse" of the body, and that when it begins to calcify and show signs of aging, this is an indication that the other organs are doing the same. However, some people, even at age ninety, show absolutely no evidence of pineal calcification. Therefore, it's hard to determine the true significance of these calcium deposits.

It seems reasonable to us that the pineal may be one of the first important parts of the body to wear out simply because it is by far the most hardworking. Throughout our lives, the pineal is a veritable powerhouse, expending a tremendous amount of energy, regulating, modulating, and keeping watch over all other systems. Anything that works this hard for this long is eventually going to "burn out," and that is what we believe happens to the pineal. The pineal begins to shrink—it loses many of its pinealocytes, the cells that produce melatonin and other compounds. Our other internal body clock, the suprachiasmatic nuclei, which transmits the light signals from the retina to the pineal, also begins to lose some of its cells, and thus may lose its influence over the pineal. As the pineal slowly wears down, it stops cycling melatonin as it once did. The body begins to run out of energy, and can no longer adapt as quickly to its environment. This, in turn, produces the cascade of events that we know of as senescence or aging.

NOT BY MELATONIN ALONE

Melatonin is the primary messenger of the pineal gland, and through melatonin the pineal performs its many jobs. Melatonin is not the only compound found in the pineal gland. Melatonin is actually synthesized from two other compounds: tryptophan, an amino acid, and serotonin, another neurotransmitter. Melatonin is produced from these compounds as the body needs it.

In addition to being the precursor to melatonin, serotonin is responsible for a wide variety of activities within the body, including sleep, smooth muscle contraction, and platelet function (platelets are a type of blood cell). An excess of serotonin (and a shortage of melatonin) has been linked to some forms of depression and mood disorders. In fact, a number of psychiatric drugs, including Prozac, are called serotonin uptake inhibitors because they maintain normal serotonin levels and stimulate the production of melatonin. (Depression is often accompanied by sleep disturbances, and antidepressants can restore normal sleep patterns.) Abnormally high levels of serotonin have been found in the spinal cords of people who have committed suicide. Although serotonin performs many vital functions in the body, a serotonin imbalance can be deadly.

One of the most intriguing new studies still in its earliest stages involves another pineal compound called epithalamin, which seems to act in many ways similar to melatonin. This research suggests that there is possibly a whole group of compounds produced by the pineal to make sure that the work gets done. Epithalamin has been isolated by scientists led by the late Vladimir Dilman at the N. N. Petrov Research Institute of Oncology, in St. Petersburg, Russia. One of the researchers, V. N. Anisimov, reported on the work of his group at the Third Stromboli Conference on Cancer and Aging.

Similar to our claims for melatonin, epithalamin has also been reported to extend life span and slow down aging in laboratory rats and mice. In animal studies, epithalamin has also been shown to shrink cancerous tumors, and to reduce injury caused by exposure to X-rays. Like melatonin, this compound increases immune function and lowers blood lipids such as cholesterol and triglycerides. What we found even more intriguing is the report that when administered to elderly female rats age sixteen to eighteen months (or about sixty in human years) who have lived long past their reproductive period, epithalamin restored fertility. Amazingly, these rats were able to conceive and produce babies. Epithalamin is now being tested on women as a potential fertility drug to extend fertility for women who are nearing menopause.

In all likelihood, epithalamin and melatonin function synergistically, that is, one enhances the action of the other. However, we really won't know how epithalamin works until more work is done on this new compound. As we mentioned earlier, one of the primary reasons we have written this book is to make people aware of the potential of these compounds, so that there will be a groundswell of support for additional research in this area.

TRH is another compound found in the pineal. We mentioned it earlier in this chapter as a means through which the pineal controls the energy supply to the cells. TRH is very important because it does so much with so little. It is a very simple molecule made up of three amino acids and is ubiquitous throughout nature. TRH is found everywhere, from a blade of grass to the cells of the human brain. Our studies have shown that TRH protects thymic function and can improve immune function, and it has been successfully used as a treatment for depression. We are particularly interested in this compound, and feel that its full potential has yet to be recognized.

Several other compounds found in the pineal are closely connected to reproduction and behavior. One of these compounds, vasopressin, is involved in the milk letdown response in nursing mothers. Just the sound of a baby's crying can promote the production of this hormone and the flow of milk. This same hormone triggers the maternal urge to cuddle and hold the baby once the child is born, helping mother and baby bond. As we noted earlier, prolactin, another hormone that has an effect similar to vasopressin's, is also present in the pineal and is also a bonding hormone. Prolactin, like several other pineal compounds, can also enhance immune function, which keeps us healthy and strong.

Scientists have only begun to seriously research the pineal gland and melatonin relatively recently. As much as we know about this gland—and we know a lot—there are still volumes yet to learn and many important discoveries yet to be made. The potential is exciting, and we relish the prospect of being involved in making some of these discoveries. In the next chapter, we will focus on how we can use melatonin to turn back the aging clock.

CHAPTER 5

Melatonin: Growing Young

Do you recall how, in the first chapter of this book, when we asked you to picture yourself in your mind's eye as an "old person," you conjured the image of someone worn, frail, and growing increasingly more debilitated with the passing years?

What if we asked you to perform the same exercise now that you know that by taking melatonin you can reset your body's aging clock? Is the image you hold in your mind now different? We hope it is.

We hope that the information we have given in these chapters about the aging clock has already succeeded in changing your attitude about aging, because thanks to what we now know about melatonin and the body's aging clock, we are the first generation that need not experience the downward spiral that has become synonymous with aging. Aging, in that sense, is a thing of the past. Indeed, our purpose in writing this book is not only to change your attitude about the future, but to actually change your future.

Ours is the first generation that need not experience senescence, the dismal physical decline now associated with old age. We are the first generation that need not resign ourselves to accepting the fate that our later years will be filled with debility and disease. Ours is the first generation that has the capacity, by resetting our aging clock, to actually prolong youthful health and vitality into our eighties, nineties, and possibly even our hundreds.

The time has come for us to stop regarding our later years as a period of winding down. By resetting our body's aging clock with melatonin, we believe it is possible not only to extend life by decades, but by healthy, youthful, productive decades. Rather than growing old, we are talking about the possibility of maintaining our youthful health and functions even as we age.

In earlier chapters, we explained that the pineal, the tiny gland embedded deep within the brain, controls the aging process. We call the pineal gland our aging clock because it is the body's timekeeper. We age because our pineal function declines over time, and as it does it produces less melatonin. This reduction in melatonin signals to the rest of the body that it is time for it to age. But if we reset our aging clock by taking melatonin, we can reverse those signals and stave off the downward spiral. Is this merely some vague and nonspecific promise of renewal? On the contrary, as you will see in the chapters that follow, the research indicates that melatonin supplementation can forestall the very real and very destructive effects of aging, including weakened immune function, cancer, sleep disorders, and heart disease.

The promise of melatonin may at first strike you as miraculous but there is nothing magical or mysterious about it. Melatonin works by restoring the function of the pineal gland, and thus it restores the balance to our body that we need to maintain the health we naturally enjoy in youth. The pineal gland is the "regulator" of the glands in our body that produce the hormones that run all our essential bodily systems. By keeping the pineal gland functioning well, melatonin helps to sustain and maintain all the different organ systems that keep the body running smoothly and efficiently. In youth our bodies work well because all our systems are working in tandem. Remember our analogy with the orchestra conductor? Without the conductor, the wind section and brass section may fall out of step and before long the harmonious music is lost.

As we age, and our pineal function declines, our central regulator loses some of its control over the various body systems. It is like an orchestra operating with a conductor who is no longer in control. Just as would happen in the case of the orchestra, without our central regulator performing at peak function, our body systems, once left to their own devices, soon fall out of sync. The disharmony that ensues leads to a gradual breakdown of the systems themselves. Melatonin supplementation can prevent this disorganized state of affairs from occurring.

We believe that melatonin supplementation works because it addresses not the symptoms but the underlying disease, which is aging itself. The positive effects of melatonin are well documented. It has been shown to bolster immune function, lower blood cholesterol levels, protect against the negative effects of stress, restore healthy sleep patterns, and help the body defend against cancer and heart disease. We want to emphasize, however, that these individual benefits are the result of melatonin's more primary and overarching function—to target the underlying conditions that give rise to these particular problems. We believe that what is truly remarkable in the discoveries regarding melatonin and the pineal gland is that we now have the key to getting ahead of the degenerative diseases normally associated with aging. By taking only a very small dose of melatonin, just enough to boost your melatonin level back to what it was when you were in your twenties, you can keep your body and each of its essential systems functioning in the synchronized manner they did in your youth. (Please refer to Chapter 14 for detailed discussion of dosage recommendations.) By supplementing melatonin after our natural production drops off, we can thereby maintain the conditions that kept us healthy, vital, and youthful in our younger years. To better understand exactly how melatonin works these wonders upon our bodies, let's take a closer look at the mechanics involved in the age-reversing properties of melatonin.

MELATONIN: THE NORMALIZER

As we have observed, the pineal gland is not just another gland; on the contrary, it is the super-gland that regulates all other glands. The pineal gland is called the regulator of the body because it helps to maintain normal hormone levels and the normal cycling of hormones. It does this by transmitting messages through its primary messenger, melatonin.

Hormones control virtually all of our bodily functions, including the maintenance of body temperature, reproduction, blood pressure, kidney function, and even the very beating of our hearts. Melatonin is a buffer hormone, because unlike other hormones that exert a direct, targeted influence on a particular organ or system, melatonin operates indirectly by modulating or fine-tuning other hormone levels. The job of melatonin is to ensure that the levels of other vital hormones stay within a normal range in response to environmental change.

As we age, the levels of many key hormones change, and this can throw our body's organ systems out of whack. This happens because the pineal gland, the regulator, begins to break down, and as a result its ability to produce melatonin begins to falter. By taking melatonin supplements, we can strengthen the functioning of the pineal gland and prevent further destruction. By restoring the pineal function, we can restore other important hormones to their youthful levels, and by doing so, we will retain the youthful state of our bodies.

The way in which melatonin helps our bodies combat the negative effects of stress is a good example. When we are under stress, our adrenal glands produce stress hormones called corticosteroids. Exposure over time to high levels of corticosteroids can cause damage to many of our organs, including the heart, the brain, and even the arteries that carry blood throughout the body. Indeed, chronic exposure to corticosteroids has been linked both to heart disease and Alzheimer's disease. When we are young and our corticosteroid levels become too high, it is melatonin that works together with other hormones to quickly bring them down to normal levels. But as we age, and our melatonin level declines, its influence on corticosteroids declines too. As a result, our corticosteroid level remains higher for longer periods of time, thus increasing our exposure to these potentially damaging hormones. By taking melatonin, we can restore corticosteroids back to healthier youthful levels. (For more on stress, see Chapter 11.)

Much of what goes wrong in old age is the effect of our hormones no longer maintaining the balance they once did. In fact the diseases that have become associated with normal aging such as diabetes and heart disease, as well as many types of cancers, are largely the result of what happens when the correct balance of hormone levels is upset. By restoring the proper hormonal balance, melatonin can help prevent many of these diseases and keep our bodies youthful.

MELATONIN: THE ANTIOXIDANT

Melatonin also helps us maintain our balance by working as an antioxidant and free-radical scavenger. You have probably heard of antioxidant vitamins, and we would not be surprised if you are already taking them yourself. You may have heard antioxidants touted as anti-aging vitamins, and, if so, you may have wondered why. The antioxidant theory of aging was proposed some four decades ago by scientist Denham Harman, who noticed that mild radiation poisoning produced symptoms that were similar to premature aging. Dr. Harman believed that aging was basically a form of "rusting," and that like an old car left out in the rain, or a cut apple left exposed to the air, our bodies can also form a kind of "rust" that prevents them from operating efficiently. He believed that exposure to radiation and other substances could accelerate this rusting.

This "rust" is caused by the most unlikely of culprits—oxygen. We know that oxygen is necessary for life, and we couldn't survive for more than a few minutes without it. Oxygen is necessary for literally every bodily function. Without it, even the simplest task would be impossible.

Oxygen is involved in metabolism, the process by which cells make energy. Energy is required for every body function from breathing to cell division to the beating of our hearts. Without energy, our bodies would simply stop working. Yet in the wrong form, oxygen can be very dangerous. In the process of making energy, however, cells can also produce substances called free radicals. Free radicals, produced in excess or inappropriately handled by the body, cause tissue damage. Cells, like everything else in the universe, are composed of smaller particles called atoms.

Each atom contains a center or nucleus that is surrounded by electrons that orbit around the cell much like the planets orbit around the sun. At times, an electron can be kicked out of its orbit. Once free, it frantically looks for another "sun" and immediately joins the orbit of another atom. When it unites with the new atom, it creates a newly energized, highly unstable atom called a free radical. The free radical is simply bursting with energy, and looks for another atom with which it can share its excess energy. In the body, free radicals transfer their energy to the cells of body tissues, and this can cause great damage.

Free radicals in excess are troublesome because they can destroy cell membranes, the protective covering of cells, and actually get into the cell nucleus, which houses DNA, the precious genetic material. Free radicals can inflict terrible damage upon DNA, and can thus impair the ability of a cell to divide and repair itself. This, in turn, can lead to a breakdown of bodily systems that will eventually result in what we know as the "aging process."

Damage inflicted by free radicals is also believed to be responsible for many other diseases, including cancer, heart disease, diabetes, Parkinson's disease, cataracts, and arthritis. When the DNA or genetic material is altered, the changes can be passed on to subsequent generations, causing birth defects.

Human beings and animals have developed mechanisms that can protect against the formation of dangerous free radicals. Our bodies naturally produce many compounds that function as antioxidants, and that prevent oxidative damage to cells; and as free-radical scavengers, they gobble up free radicals before they can wreak their cellular havoc. Antioxidants found in the body include vitamin E, glutathione, selenium, and vitamin C. As we age, we may need more antioxidants and free-radical scavengers, and we are more prone to oxidative damage. One way to avoid free-radical formation is to limit exposure to substances that promote them. Radiation, ultraviolet light, cigarette smoke, smog, and polyunsaturated fats are all substances that are believed to trigger free-radical production in the body. The excess accumulation in the body of metals such as iron can also promote the formation of free radicals.

Another way to control the formation of free radicals is to take antioxidant supplements, such as vitamins C and E, selenium, and the carotenes, which may help restore the proper balance of antioxidants and free-radical scavengers. We believe that melatonin will soon be added to this list because recent studies have demonstrated that melatonin may also be a potent antioxidant and free-radical scavenger. At the Third Stromboli Conference on Aging and Cancer, Dr. Russell Reiter presented a provocative paper entitled "Melatonin As a Free Radical Scavenger: Implications for Aging and Age-Related Diseases." The paper is published in *The Aging Clock* (edited by Walter Pierpaoli, William Regelson, and Nicola Fabris), the bound proceedings of the conference that were published by the New York Academy of Sciences. Dr. Reiter tested the effect of melatonin against a potent carcinogen that is well known to damage DNA by stimulating the production of free radicals. He found that melatonin was able to neutralize the carcinogen and thwart its destructive effects, proving that melatonin is indeed a free-radical scavenger.

This study also suggested how melatonin may work within the cell. Melatonin is lipid-soluble, which means it passes very easily through cell membranes— the protective surface outside of the cells that allow certain substances in, but block the entry of others. Melatonin, in particular, seems to have an affinity for the cell nucleus, the place within the cell where the precious DNA is stored. Dr. Reiter believes that melatonin's role within the nucleus is primarily to protect the DNA. We find this explanation intriguing and imaginative, and we have even tested melatonin's potential as a free radical in our own laboratories. One of our colleagues has shown that in a tissue culture model, at the right concentration, melatonin can protect liver cells against oxidative injury. This study showed that melatonin as an antioxidant was no better than vitamin E, another potent oxidant and free-radical scavenger. Although we also believe that melatonin may function as an antioxidant, we do not believe that this one role should overshadow the other incredibly important place it has in the body. If you step back and look at the big picture, melatonin's role is far greater than that of just another antioxidant.

MELATONIN: IT'S ALL ABOUT ENERGY

We believe another one of melatonin's job may be to protect the body's energy system, which is critical for our survival. Our bodies require energy or fuel to keep them going. A body that runs out of fuel can't function at peak capacity and eventually winds down and wears out. The pineal gland and melatonin may operate in tandem to control the energy system that fuels the cells and keeps the body functioning well. Without the proper amount of energy, all of our body systems are thrown out of whack.

The pineal gland controls the production of a hormone called TRH (thyrotropin-releasing hormone), which stimulates the production of TSH (thyroid-stimulating hormone), which, in turn, as its name implies, triggers the production of thyroid hormone. TSH stimulates the thyroid to secrete two hormones,

T_3 and T_4. Melatonin regulates the breakdown of T_4 into T_3, a much more energetic form of thyroid hormone, and by doing so influences the flow of energy to all of the body organs and glands, including the pineal gland itself.

What is this energy for? We need energy to run our body systems and to provide the heat to keep us warm, but we also need energy to produce more energy. Energy is created in the cells by microscopic structures called mitochondria. Mitochondria produce ATP (adenosine triphosphate), which is quite literally the fuel that drives the body. As we age, our mitochondria begin to age too. They lose their shape and structure, become hardened or calcified, and are no longer able to repair themselves or make new mitochondria. As the mitochondria "burn out," they produce less and less ATP, and so the body has less fuel or energy to run on. This is why a young person can race up a flight of steps two at a time, but an elderly person may need to stop every two steps for a rest. This is not just a problem of poor circulation. Quite simply, without energy, we tire more easily.

Oxygen is essential for the production of ATP, and it is burned up in the process. When the production of ATP by the mitochondria slows down, however, there is an excess of oxygen, which can lead to the formation of free radicals. As we have just seen, free radicals can damage tissues and organ systems.

This brings us back to melatonin. As we said earlier, melatonin metabolizes thyroid hormone into a more potent form that provides the cells with more energy. Therefore, by providing energy to the mitochondria to produce more ATP, melatonin may prevent the formation of free radicals in all organs and glands of the body, including the critical pineal gland.

As the regulator of all other glands, the pineal is one of the most active glands in the body, constantly creating and consuming energy. If the pineal is to continue to function at a youthful level, it also needs energy. It must produce enough ATP to sustain it. If the pineal gland has enough ATP, it can continue its regulatory role in an efficient manner.

Once the pineal gland begins to break down, however, the energy system of the body is slowly thrown out of kilter. Pineal function begins to decline when the mitochondria in the cells of the pineal run out of energy and can no longer make enough ATP. Instead, they produce another compound called pyrophosphate, which can actually do damage to the body. Pyrophosphate binds or links up with calcium, which is present in all cells, and forms calcium salt. As the pineal ages, it calcifies and becomes hard. Once the pineal calcifies, its production of melatonin declines. When the levels of melatonin drop, the levels of other important hormones are altered, including thyroid hormone, and this results in less energy being made available to the cells of other body organs. Without enough energy, the mitochondria in the cells of other organs stop producing enough ATP, and begin to produce the chemical that promotes calcification. For example, calcium deposits in blood vessels can cause atherosclerosis or hardening of the arteries, which hampers the flow of blood and causes a heart attack or stroke. Calcium deposits have been found in other organs, including the brain and the heart.

As we have seen, the calcification process that begins in the pineal may spread throughout the body, causing the slow destruction of every cell and eventually every organ system. Simply put, when the pineal can no longer do its job, it results in the breakdown of mitochondria throughout the body, the powerhouses of the cells that regulate energy. When the mitochondria break down, this causes a chain reaction throughout the body that leads to the eventual collapse of all other organ systems.

In fact, many leading researchers in the field of aging now believe that a breakdown in the function of the mitochondria is the primary cause of most diseases of aging, including Alzheimer's disease, Parkinson's disease, and cancer. We believe that we are aging because the pineal gland is breaking down, which in turn causes the slowing down of the mitochondria. When the pineal gland can no longer do its job, every cell in the body goes awry, including the mitochondria. When the pineal gland breaks down, we begin to age, and this is what makes us vulnerable to disease.

THE ZINC/MELATONIN CONNECTION

We've shown the different ways in which melatonin can rejuvenate the body. Melatonin may exert its age-reversing effects in yet another way in another part of the body.

Melatonin is not only produced by the pineal gland. High concentrations of melatonin—even higher than in the pineal gland—have been found in the gastrointestinal (GI) system, known as the gut. Why are there such high amounts of melatonin in the gut or GI tract? Once again, we refer back to melatonin's role as the body's "normalizer." During digestion, food must be broken down and absorbed by the body. As it is being broken down, food must pass through the digestive tract with appropriate speed so that its nutrients can be fully absorbed. Melatonin appears to have a calming effect on the digestive tract, which may slow down the digestive process in order to give our bodies enough time to utilize the important vitamins, minerals, and other nutrients found in food. As we age, we lose the ability to absorb nutrients from our food. This, of course, may lead to vitamin and mineral deficiencies that result in damage to bodily functions. Older people typically have lower levels of many important vitamins and minerals. Melatonin supplements, by increasing our ability to absorb vitamins and minerals, may prevent that damage and thus help turn back another symptom of aging. Melatonin may also protect the liver and gut from the damaging carcinogenic action of free radicals in our food.

This reasoning is supported by the fact that melatonin aids the absorption of one key mineral in particular. Throughout this book we refer to the zinc/melatonin connection, the fact that studies have shown that melatonin can help normalize blood zinc levels. This is of particular importance to older people.

Zinc is one mineral that is often deficient in older people no matter how carefully or well they eat. A deficiency in zinc has been linked to a number of age-related problems, including loss of taste, loss of smell, and prostate problems in men. Zinc is instrumental in the functioning of the immune system, which as we discussed, declines as we age. It has been documented that zinc supplements can perk up the immune system of people over age seventy, as shown by an increase in T cells, which help fight infection. Interestingly, as we'll discuss in greater detail in the chapter on melatonin's role in enhancing immunity, zinc and melatonin have similar effects on the immune system. A decline in zinc levels may also be responsible for one of the leading causes of blindness among the elderly.

It seems to us that the presence of melatonin in the gut is connected with the absorption of zinc, and specifically that melatonin participates in the synthesis of molecules that are involved in zinc transport, or the movement of zinc in and out of the cells. Here again we see melatonin operating to restore the normal, youthful balance of a critical body system.

In Part One we have explained the promise that melatonin holds as an age-reversing agent that can prevent the devastating physical and mental decline associated with aging. We have seen how in literally hundreds of different ways—some subtle, some blatant—melatonin is constantly correcting, regulating, and normalizing all of the body's activities. It keeps the blood flowing through our hearts, it keeps our hormone levels normal, it protects us from the damage inflicted by free radicals, it keeps our reproductive systems vital and strong and our immune systems "battle ready." Whether we are young or older, melatonin helps us adapt and respond to our external and internal environments.

One of melatonin's greatest promises is its ability to keep us disease-free. Maintaining health is essential to maintaining a youthful body. As we turn to Part Two, we will be looking at the role of melatonin as a disease-fighting hormone. As you will see, melatonin appears to play an important role in the prevention and possible treatment of many different diseases, including cancer and heart disease. As a prelude to that, however, we will in the next chapter look at the fundamentals of the body's disease-fighting system—the immune system—and how melatonin can keep it vigilant and strong.

PART TWO

Nature's Disease-Fighting Hormone

CHAPTER 6

The Immune System: Nature's Own Bodyguard

THE PROMISE OF MELATONIN:

- Strengthens your immune system
- Fights against disease
- Maintains youthful health and vigor

When we refer to melatonin as a disease-fighting hormone, we're not just talking about some new treatment or cure for one particular disease or even several diseases. The implications for melatonin are far more profound.

We believe that aging itself is a disease that drains our vitality, and shortens our lives. Ideally, the best way to protect against the various diseases associated with our later years, such as cancer, heart disease, and diabetes, is to prevent the destructive effects of aging and to vigorously defend our bodies before disease can take hold. We believe it is possible to do this by taking melatonin. Restoring melatonin to the levels of our youth should not only significantly extend our lives, but also keep our bodies more resistant to disease and, therefore, healthier. What that means is that we can remain physically strong and retain our vigor not just in youth, but throughout our entire lives. As far as we are concerned, extending life is meaningless, if we can't also live those extra years in a strong, vital body. It is not enough to simply add decades. They must be decades that are worth living.

As we explained in Part One, melatonin can rejuvenate pineal function, and by doing so can help bolster and preserve the efficiency of each primary organ system in the body. Most importantly, it can boost immunity and thus strengthen our resistance against infection and cancer. It can also help keep our cholesterol levels normal and our hearts strong. It may even be useful for the treatment of problems such as Down syndrome, the most common form of congenital mental retardation, and Alzheimer's disease, and even AIDS.

In the next section, you will read about the many potential medical uses for melatonin currently under investigation by scientists across the globe. We're not giving you this information so that you can self-diagnose or self-prescribe. If you have a medical problem, you should be under a doctor's supervision. What you are about to learn should be used in conjunction with conventional therapy.

THE IMMUNE SYSTEM: NATURE'S OWN BODYGUARD

The immune system is our body's defense mechanism against disease. It is a highly sophisticated network of fighter cells that seek out and destroy viruses, bacteria, precancerous and cancer cells, and other invader organisms that can do us harm. The immune system also has to know when not to fight back. For example, it must know how to identify our own body tissues so that it does not wage war against our own organs. It also must allow us to digest and absorb food, which is full of foreign proteins and other substances. If the immune system did not know when to call off its troops, our bodies would reject the food we eat and we would starve.

As we age, our immune system ages too, and it becomes weaker and less effective. Although we produce the same number of disease-fighting cells, these cells do not work as well. That is why older people are more prone to illnesses of all kinds. A child can quickly shake off a cold, but what begins as a sniffle and remains a cold in a child, may develop into a bad case of pneumonia in a grandparent. The older we are, the greater our risk of developing many different forms of cancer.

As we age, we are also more vulnerable to disorders of the immune system itself. These are called autoimmune diseases. When they occur, our immune cells become confused, and begin to attack our body's own tissue. This is precisely what occurs in the case of rheumatoid arthritis, a common problem among older people.

This gradual breakdown in our immune system need not occur. It happens because our pineal glands are aging, and they are issuing orders to other body systems to age as well. Our studies suggest that by taking melatonin, we can keep our immune system functioning at peak capacity, just like it did when we were young. Melatonin works because it resets our aging clocks—our pineal glands—so that our hormones and the systems that they regulate are also reset at more youthful, healthier levels. Therefore, the immune system of an older person who is taking melatonin is as strong as a much younger immune system, and that person is bound to stay healthier.

The Melatonin Miracle

In this section, we will describe how the immune system operates, how it is affected by the amount of melatonin secreted by the pineal gland, and how, by melatonin supplementation, we can slow down the aging of the immune system. We will explain how, by preserving the strength and resilience of the pineal gland and the immune system, we help protect our bodies from diseases and their degenerative effects. We will show that the best way to fight disease is to prevent it, and that the pineal gland and melatonin can play a vital role in this effort.

As we have said in previous chapters of this book, but it bears repeating here, we regard aging as the ultimate disease, and we have also come to recognize that the effect of disease is, in turn, rapid aging. To better understand what we mean, consider this: A twenty-five-year-old with AIDS has many of the same health problems as an eighty-year-old whose immune system has been weakened by aging. In the case of the twenty-five-year-old, disease has ravaged the immune system, causing, in effect, rapid aging. In the case of the eighty-year-old, aging has weakened the immune system, causing disease, which in turn causes the body to degrade further. We believe that we can intervene and disrupt this aging→disease→aging cycle by strengthening the pineal function and supplementing its melatonin output. Thus, by strengthening the immune system and its disease-fighting power, we stave off both the major cause and the major effect of what we know as aging.

In many ways, the immune system acts as a mirror of the aging process itself. As our body's prime defender, the immune system must be able to distinguish our own cells from undesirable, alien cells; it must protect "self" from "nonself." But, as we get older, our immune system becomes "forgetful" and makes mistakes as a consequence. The reason is that as we age we lose some of the cells in the immune system that are responsible for memory, and that are programmed to distinguish friend from foe. As these cells disappear, the immune system no longer remembers who we are and what makes each of us unique. When this happens, our aging immune system may allow enemy cells to flourish, and as a result we may contract a bacterial or viral infection that we might have easily been able to ward off in our youth. What is equally devastating is when our own immune cells become so confused that they begin to attack our very own tissues and organs, causing the very illnesses the system was designed to prevent. It is as if the "eyes" of our immune system are clouding and becoming unable to distinguish good cells from bad cells. The result of this system breakdown is that we lose some of the integrity of our cellular identity; our "selfness" declines. It is nature's way of slowly writing us out of the play of life to make room for stronger, healthier creatures.

This loss of identity and the tangible physical loss that accompanies it extend far beyond the immune system. There is a psychological or spiritual component to this loss of identity that is every bit as real. Picture in your mind the "elderly" people you have known, and you will immediately see what we mean. As people grow older and their bodies begin to fail, they often suffer a loss of sense of self that is manifested in depression and a lack of interest in the very things that had once been so important to them, and they become increasingly isolated from the world around them. They become removed from the mainstream of life, grow old in isolation, and they seem to progressively disappear. While we believe that this phenomenon is in part due to the way certain societies treat their elders, we also believe that what is going on inside the body is responsible. Degenerative changes in the body and the brain work together to accelerate this loss of identity.

Melatonin works to prevent the loss of identity, on both the physical and psychic levels. As we will show in this chapter, melatonin can help keep an aging immune system functioning with more of the strength and vigor it manifests in our youth. We believe that accumulating years in a healthy, strong, "young" body will not be the same experience as senescing. This was once thought to be the inevitable and necessary condition of our later decades, but such conventional thinking must now be reconsidered. To the extent that melatonin helps us retain our health and powers as we age, it also enables us to maintain a strong identity and a firm sense of self.

The key to maintaining identity is to maintain a well-functioning, "smart" immune system that can distinguish between good and bad cells and respond quickly to whatever challenges that may come its way. In this chapter, we're going to focus on how the immune system works, and how melatonin can make it work even better.

The immune system is, perhaps, the most complicated, finely tuned system in the body. We are just beginning to unravel its vast secrets, but there is much more scientists still do not understand. Viruses such as HIV, the one that causes AIDS, are able to enter the body and subvert the entire immune system in ways that we do not yet fully comprehend, and that also leave us helpless to respond.

The immune system is comprised of many different components that perform many different tasks. The main cells of the immune system are white blood cells called lymphocytes. T cells are a particular type of lymphocyte produced in the thymus, a small gland located at the sternum in front of the breastbone. T cells help fight against cancer, certain types of bacteria and viruses, and fungal infections like *Candida albicans,* which can cause troublesome yeast infections in women. T cells are also responsible for the delayed skin reactions that occur after exposure to bacteria. For example, most if not all of you have probably had a skin test for tuberculosis. The physician scratches the skin with a needle contaminated with a minute quantity of the tuberculosis bacillus, the bacterium that causes this disease. If sometime in your life you were exposed to the tuberculosis bacterium, small bumps will appear on the test site a few days later, indicating that the test result is positive. These bumps are caused by angry T cells, which, having recognized a known offender, the TB bacillus, rush to the test site to protect you against further injury. T cells, which also protect the body from foreign proteins, are also involved in the rejection of transplanted organs. When transplant patients receive new organs, for example, they must be given drugs that will dampen their immune response, so that their bodies do not reject the transplanted organ, which is going to be perceived as a foreign invader.

An army of well-functioning T cells is critical for our survival. When we age, our T cells become less effective, and as a result, we are more prone to illness. It is also the loss of two kinds of T cells that causes AIDS. One is the type of T cell that protects cells against invasion by viruses and bacteria. The other is the type of T cell that circulates throughout the bloodstream looking for potential troublemakers, functioning as the immune system's cop on the beat. When these crucial T cells are lost, the immune system is virtually knocked out, and the body is unable to fend off disease. As we discuss more fully in the section on AIDS, the effect of this disease, in a very real sense, is to prematurely "age" its victims.

Other lymphocytes, called B lymphocytes or B

cells, produce proteins called antibodies or immunoglobulins. When a foreign substance or antigen is introduced into the body, B cells quickly respond by making antibodies, which attach themselves to the invaders. If this doesn't stop the infection, other immune cells will join in the attack. The body can make thousands of different antibodies, each designed to search out and destroy a specific antigen.

Antibodies have an excellent memory, which is why in some cases we can develop immunity to specific diseases after we have had them. A familiar case in point is chicken pox. Most people only get chicken pox once in their lives, and if they are exposed to the chicken pox virus later, they are usually immune to it. The reason is that antibodies that were manufactured in response to the first exposure remain in the bloodstream, continually on watch for the return of the chicken pox antigen. If it appears, the antibodies strike. We do not have to develop the full-blown disease to gain immunity from a virus. For example, when you receive a vaccination against a particular disease, such as measles, the B cells respond by producing specific antibodies against the measles virus. If the measles virus later enters the body in an active state, those previously formed antibodies will attack the virus and, with the help of other cells, destroy it.

In addition to fighting against infection, one of the primary functions of the immune system is also to maintain a lookout for signs of cancerous cells, and to destroy them before they can do any harm. Back in 1970, cancer researcher F. M. Burnet coined the word "immunosurveillance" to describe how the immune system closely monitors the body for potential cancers and, upon identifying them, quickly eradicates them. This process occurs continuously in our bodies, and many scientists believe that cancer is actually a disease caused by a malfunctioning immune surveillance system. Many medical researchers believe that keeping our immune system strong may be the best way to effectively prevent cancer, and we discuss this in our chapter on cancer.

There are other kinds of immune cells that also play a major role in keeping us well. These cells include macrophages, which are large cells that gobble up foreign material found in the body. Some macrophages reside in the lungs, where they ingest inhaled dust, while others occupy the bone marrow, connective tissue, and the lining of major organs. When a part of the body becomes infected, macrophages are let loose into the bloodstream, through which they travel to the point of infection and do their work.

Between the ages of seventy and eighty, we typically experience a dramatic decline in immune function, as we have already mentioned. Although we have as many T cells as we had when we were younger, they are no longer as effective. By this age, no more than half of our aging T cells are still capable of responding to an antigen (enemy), and for some people that number falls as low as 20 percent. Why does this happen? This decline occurs because the memory cells of the immune system cease to recognize potential troublemakers and therefore do not respond quickly by dispatching its army of antibodies to disarm them. The consequence is that we get sicker more often.

Some T cells are known as helper cells, and, as their name suggests, they help wage the battle against infection. Other T cells are known as suppressor cells, and these cells actually can suppress an attack by the immune system. For example, suppressor cells keep helper cells from destroying the body's own tissue, and a malfunction of these cells may cause autoimmune diseases. In many older people, for reasons still being researched, the suppressor cells cease to function. In this case, their body's own antibodies begin to attack their own cells. This in turn can trigger the onset of any number of autoimmune diseases, including rheumatoid arthritis, Sjögren's syndrome (dry mouth, dry eye), and thyroid diseases. Some researchers feel that this friendly fire may not be the fault of the immune system, but actually a result of a slight change in the way proteins are produced by our bodies that often occurs as we age. Although the resulting new proteins are similar to the original ones, they look strange and foreign to the antibodies, which promptly attack them.

Our immune system is also affected by environmental factors. For example, malnutrition or viruses such as influenza and HIV can seriously weaken the immune system's capacity to defend against disease. Malnutrition may be one reason why infection is rampant in parts of the world where the population is poorly nourished. We also know that deficiencies in key vitamins and minerals can trigger disease. A deficiency in vitamin C, for example, may cause a decrease in T cells, which, as we have seen, are the disease-killing cells of the immune system. The kinds of foods we consume may also affect immune function. For example, animal studies have shown that a high-fat diet can significantly weaken immune response by impairing T cell function. Not surprisingly, some studies have linked a diet high in fat to an increased incidence of certain forms of cancer in humans.

This quick overview helps to make apparent how the immune system plays a critical role in keeping us disease-free and healthy. It also demonstrates that as we age the immune system progressively decays, which results in diminished health. What we have seen about the immune system is that when we are in youthful health, it ensures its efficiency by targeting its enemies on many fronts. When we are under attack, our immune system dispatches its army of T cells, B cells, surveillance cells, antibodies, and other warriors to defend the fortress against invaders. How, then, do we protect this vital system from growing old? The answer is melatonin.

Our studies, confirmed by others, have shown that melatonin can have a significant positive effect on immune function, on a variety of fronts. In the following section, we will explain how melatonin can keep your immune system working at peak capacity.

MELATONIN RESTORES THYMUS FUNCTION

Why do we lose our ability to fight disease as we age? We believe that one reason is that, as we age, we lose our thymus gland, the small gland located behind the breastbone from which the powerful T cells are stored and controlled. The thymus weighs about half an ounce at birth and doubles in size by puberty. After that, it begins to shrink and is replaced by fatty tissue. As this happens, our T cells gradually lose their fighting power. As we explained in Chapters 2 and 3, we have found that when melatonin was added to the nighttime drinking water of older mice, melatonin not only significantly extended their life span, but also kept the mice disease-free by improving their immune response. Here is what we found:

- Melatonin increased the weight of the thymus.
- Melatonin increased the activity of thymus cells, indicating that they were more actively producing T cell lymphocytes.
- Melatonin restored skin sensitivity to known allergens, a sign that the "memory" of the T cells had

been restored. In other words, the cells were better able to identify potential enemies and take action to repel them.

Moreover, in a subsequent experiment, when we transplanted peak-melatonin-producing pineal glands from young mice into the bodies of old mice, and transplanted low-melatonin-producing pineal glands from old mice into the bodies of young mice, the influence of the pineal on the thymus gland was even more dramatic. The thymus glands of the old mice who had received the young pineals had regenerated, whereas the thymus glands of the young mice who had received the old pineals had withered. Their aging was accelerated!

MELATONIN STRENGTHENS ANTIBODY RESPONSE

As we discussed in the overview on the immune system, when our immune systems age, they become less able to manufacture antibodies—the "troops" that are specifically designed to attack invading organisms such as viruses and bacteria. The result is that, as we age, we become more vulnerable to infection. Our research has shown that melatonin supplementation can reverse this downward slide.

In one experiment, we tested how a loss of melatonin would affect the body's ability to manufacture these disease-fighting antibodies. We gave mice drugs that had the effect of preventing their pineal glands from producing the usual nighttime surge in melatonin. In each case, we found that the decline in melatonin level resulted in severe suppression of the immune system, and a marked decline in the ability of the mice to produce antibodies. However, when we gave the mice melatonin to restore their normal nighttime peak levels, their immune system bounced back.

In another experiment, we investigated whether melatonin could improve the immune system's ability to produce antibodies against a foreign invader. In this experiment, two groups of mice received injections of a foreign protein, red blood cells from sheep. The dosage was just enough to immunize the mice, that is, to trigger the production of antibodies against the protein without making the animals sick. Once antibodies are produced against a protein, the body has a built-in memory for fighting against this invader the next time it encounters it. One group of mice was then given melatonin supplements for seven days following the immunization, and the other group was not. Several weeks later we gave both groups another injection of sheep blood cells. As we had expected, the mice that had received the melatonin supplements showed a much stronger immune response against the foreign protein than the untreated mice, which proved that melatonin had strengthened their antibody response.

This experiment demonstrated that melatonin was able to improve the antibody response against a specific antigen. This is important for several reasons. First, if melatonin can enhance the response to immunization, then there may be good reason to routinely administer melatonin along with standard immunizations. Certainly, more research is warranted here. Second, the loss of antibody response is a major problem of aging—perhaps *the* major problem, in that our inability to wage a strong attack against an invader weakens us and leaves us susceptible to a myriad of health problems. If we can reverse the diminishing efficiency of immune response, or prevent the decline from happening in the first place, we believe we can keep our immune system in a perpetually youthful state. The more youthful our immune system, the less susceptible we are to disease. The less disease we suffer, the less we age. Thus, by strengthening our antibodies, melatonin can stave off a major cause and a major effect of aging.

MELATONIN HELPS FIGHT AGAINST VIRUSES

Movies such as *Outbreak* and books like *The Hot Zone* underscore our morbid fascination with viruses, those microscopic disease-causing agents that are capable of striking terror in our hearts because they are capable of doing so much damage to our bodies. Unlike bacteria, a virus can only reproduce when it comes in contact with another living cell. When they do come in contact with another living cell they attach themselves to it, and quite literally take over the workings of the cell. When this happens, the cell begins to manufacture more of the virus, and the process repeats. In most cases, a virus is no match for our T cells, and eventually it is beaten down. Some viruses, however, are harder to destroy than others, and some, such as HIV, defeat the immune system before the immune system can defeat the virus. Unlike bacteria, which can be killed by antibiotics, drugs are largely ineffective against viruses. If a virus is found to be the cause of a particular disease, however, it can be isolated and made into a vaccine, a low dose or weakened form of the virus that is just strong enough to trigger the production of antibodies. In this way, the body can develop immunity without actually contracting the virus.

Occasionally, science has been able to develop vaccines to protect us from viruses, but in a world filled with many thousands of old, new, or mutating viruses, vaccines are not a complete solution. Therefore, any substance that helps the immune system ward off a dangerous virus is of great value, and melatonin is such a substance.

In one study, we injected mice with encephalomyo-carditis virus, a lethal virus that causes an infection of the lining of the heart. We then administered melatonin to the infected mice. We found that melatonin decreased the rate of mortality associated with the virus, and also suppressed the potentially damaging inflammatory response that is triggered by the virus. Based on this study, and our other studies that show that melatonin can heighten immune response, we believe that melatonin may knock out some viruses before they can inflict their harm.

THE THYROID AND IMMUNITY

The thyroid gland lies at the base of the neck, above the thymus. It produces hormones that can increase the production of T cells, and therefore the thyroid is important to the maintenance of a strong immune system. In fact, people with low thyroid function are more prone to infection. Our studies have shown that both melatonin supplementation in the drinking water of aging mice, and the transplantation of a young pineal gland into an older mouse can rejuvenate thyroid function. Since an improvement in thyroid function has an overall positive effect on immunity, this is yet another example of how melatonin helps the immune system do its job better.

MELATONIN BLOCKS DAMAGE TO THE IMMUNE SYSTEM CAUSED BY STRESS

Stress can have a devastating effect on the immune system. People who are under physical or mental stress are more vulnerable to disease, and more likely to fall prey to a viral or bacterial infection that, under less stressful circumstances, they might be able to shake off. It's been well documented that the caring spouses of people with Alzheimer's disease have depressed immune systems, and it's been suggested that the stress of ministering to a chronically sick relative is responsible for the decline. Other studies have shown that when astronauts return from a space flight, during their first four days back on earth the ability of their T cells to respond to disease is severely impaired. Space flight is a risky business. Clearly the stress of the job is taking its toll on the astronaut's immune system.

Stressful situations stimulate the production of corticosteroids by the adrenal glands, which are located on top of the kidneys and are part of the endocrine system. Corticosteroids are important because they raise blood sugar levels, giving us a burst of energy that is needed to cope with a stressful situation. For example, if you're crossing a street and you see a car coming at you, you feel a surge of fear, but you also feel pumped for action. Your thoughts race, your heart starts to pound, and a sudden burst of corticosteroids, adrenaline as well as other stress hormones, helps you move your legs faster to get out of harm's way. Similarly, when your body is threatened not by an oncoming car but by a viral or bacterial infection, this too is a highly stressful situation for your body systems, and, as a result, you produce more corticosteroids. For example, AIDS patients, as might be expected, often have extraordinarily high levels of corticosteroids. Corticosteroids, however, also have a downside, particularly if you are constantly churning them out. These hormones can dampen the immune response by blocking the production of disease-fighting antibodies, hampering the manufacture of T cells and preventing immune cells from entering the inflamed tissues where they are needed. Over time, stress can also cause significant damage to muscle and connective tissue, parts of the brain, particularly those that control memory, and other body organs. Chronic exposure to corticosteroids due to stress may even be a factor in autoimmune diseases.

There is an antidote to the damage inflicted by these corticosteroids, and it is melatonin. Our experiments have shown that when mice who are subjected to stress are also given melatonin supplements, the effects of overproduction of corticosteroids are moderated. Their thymus glands do not shrivel up, or "age," and they continue to produce normal levels of disease-fighting T cells. Thus, melatonin supplements can help counteract some of the most debilitating health effects of stress. (For more detailed information on stress and melatonin, see Chapter 11.)

THE ZINC CONNECTION

As baby boomers begin to age, we predict there is going to be a lot more attention paid to zinc in general, and its interaction with melatonin in particular. Zinc, a mineral, is a major player in the immune system, and studies have shown that many older people are deficient in this mineral. In some cases, this may result because they are not getting enough zinc in their diet. But in other cases, it most likely results from the fact that although their diets contain sufficient zinc, their bodies are not absorbing it properly. A zinc-deficient diet in older animals can impair T cell function and result in low levels of thyroid hormone, both of which can inflict serious harm to the immune system.

Studies have shown that zinc supplements can produce many of the same beneficial effects on the immune system as melatonin, such as rejuvenating thymic function and generally improving immune response.

We are exploring the possibility of a melatonin/zinc connection in which melatonin is instrumental in the transport and absorption of zinc in the body. We have good reason to suspect this to be the case. Our studies with our colleagues in Ancona have shown that melatonin supplements or pineal transplantation from a young mouse to an old mouse can restore low zinc plasma levels to normal values. As we have pointed out in previous chapters, giving an old mouse a new pineal is a way of increasing its melatonin levels and restoring them to their youthful levels.

The decline in zinc blood levels as we age is believed to be responsible for the loss of many functions that typically occur in aging. For example, if you are zinc-deficient, you lose your ability to taste food, and not so coincidentally, the loss of taste is a common problem of the elderly. Male sexual function is also linked to zinc, and that, too, can suffer with age. In fact, there is more zinc in the prostate than any other part of a man's body. If melatonin supplements can normalize the zinc levels as we put on years, many of the problems associated with aging, including impaired immune function, and prostate hypertrophy in men, may be put on hold.

SLEEP AND IMMUNITY

Have you ever noticed how, after you've missed too many hours of sleep, you seem to catch every cold that comes your way? Several studies have linked sleep deprivation to a sharp decline in immune function. For example, one study performed at the San Diego Veterans Affairs Medical Center observed twenty-three healthy men, ages twenty-two to sixty-one, for four nights in a sleep laboratory. On the third night, the men were denied sleep between the hours of 3 and 7 A.M., forfeiting about half a good night's sleep. The morning after the sleep deprivation, eighteen of the twenty-three men showed a noticeable decline in activity among the type of T cells that combat viral infections. Fortunately, after a good night's sleep, the activity level of these T cells was restored. The researchers could not say for sure whether this drop in natural killer cells would result in an increased susceptibility to viral infection, but they suggested that it could.

The researchers were at a loss to explain why sleep deprivation would have such an immediate and noticeable effect on immune function. Since melatonin blood levels peak during the night, during sleep, it seems obvious to us that lack of sleep may result in a drop or alteration of circulating melatonin, which could contribute to the decline in immunity.

In this chapter, we have shown how melatonin, by bolstering our immune system, can help prevent many of the diseases associated with old age. Indeed, we regard this as melatonin's single most important contribution as a disease-fighting hormone. The downward spiral of physical decline associated with growing old, which has become known as senescence,

Melatonin for a Strong Immune System

By taking melatonin supplements, we can boost our immune function, which otherwise declines with age. Our age-reversal therapy works in large part because melatonin supplements can help restore the immune system to its youthful capacity. Since our melatonin levels begin to decline in our forties, we need to replenish our natural melatonin supply and thereby help to restore our immune function to its youthful level. As we have stated throughout this book, it is our belief that the best way to fight disease is through prevention, and a strong immune system is our best defense. The dosage of melatonin that is right for you will depend on your age. Turn to Chapter 14 for details and instructions.

is the primary cause of all other diseases that strike in our later years. By maintaining the body in a youthful state with melatonin, we will be able to prevent the dismal decline that is characterized by physical degeneration and debilitating illness. With melatonin, we should be able to fortify ourselves against the diseases of aging. With melatonin, we do not have to live out our later years in an increasingly sick and broken body. Melatonin is not only an age-reversing hormone that will add years to your life, but what is even more exciting is the promise of adding healthy years.

In the next few chapters, we will describe the work of researchers around the world who are exploring different ways to utilize melatonin's disease-fighting properties for the treatment and prevention of common diseases such as cancer and heart disease. We will also show how melatonin may prove to be a useful therapy for a wide range of other diseases, including Alzheimer's, AIDS, eye disorders, diabetes, Down's syndrome, and other common ailments.

CHAPTER 7

Melatonin: A Powerful Protector and Treatment Against Cancer

THE PROMISE OF MELATONIN:

- Bolsters body's ability to search and destroy cancer cells
- Helps protect against breast and prostate cancer
- Helps body defend against cancer-causing agents
- Prevents damage to cells by free radicals

Within the past decade, a great deal of attention has been focused on compounds that are potential cancer fighters. We have heard, most recently, beta-carotene, vitamin C, shark cartilage, garlic, and dehydroepiandrosterone (DHEA) touted as weapons du jour in the war against cancer. Ironically, very little has been said to date about melatonin, and yet this hormone may hold great promise.

Nature's Disease-Fighting Hormone

As we will show in this chapter, melatonin operates as a potent cancer fighter in many ways. We will discuss important research studies that have shown that melatonin can play a role both in the treatment of cancer and in improving the quality of the lives of cancer patients.

The very real benefits of melatonin as an aid in the treatment of cancer notwithstanding, we believe melatonin's greatest value as a true disease-fighting hormone is in its ability to prevent the onset of diseases such as cancer. That is why we've devoted a great deal of time to explaining the importance of the immune system, and how the pineal gland and melatonin help keep the immune system running efficiently. As we age, the pineal begins to fail and melatonin levels drop, our immune systems decline, and we are left weak and vulnerable to disease. Nowhere is this more apparent than in the case of cancer. It is no coincidence that the risk of developing cancer rises exponentially with age. The longer we live, the more likely it is that we will develop cancer. Cancer occurs because of a breakdown in the function of the immune system; if we can keep our immune systems strong and resilient, we can remain cancer-free. We can begin to do this by reconstituting the youthful function of our pineal glands through melatonin supplementation.

The cancer-fighting properties of melatonin were first identified nearly five decades ago, when an Australian cancer specialist named K. W. Starr reported that he had used melatonin successfully to control sarcomas, a kind of tumor that grows in the bone, muscle, or connective tissue. Starr did not publish articles in any of the well-known journals of the day, and although Bill took note of it for his own research, it received little attention in the scientific world. As far as we know, until recently no one else has pursued

Starr's research, and, when he disappeared from the scene, so did his work.

Fifty years later, melatonin is now being rediscovered by oncologists who are reexamining its potential as a cancer treatment. Their interest is long overdue. In the Western world, cancer is a virtual epidemic. Estimates are that one out of three Americans will get cancer sometime in their lifetime. By the next century, that number will soar to one out of two. There isn't a family in the United States that will not be affected by this disease. Some forms of cancer—for reasons we don't quite understand—are particularly prevalent. Nearly everyone reading this book probably knows a woman who has had breast cancer, and our guess is many of you probably know several women who have had this disease. This is not surprising. According to the American Cancer Society, one out of eight women will eventually get breast cancer, and that number seems to be rising. More than forty-six thousand women die of breast cancer each year. Also disturbing is the fact that breast cancer is not the leading cause of cancer deaths among women; thanks in large part to cigarette smoking, lung cancer is.

This is not to suggest that men have been spared by the cancer epidemic. Among men over age fifty, one out of eleven will get cancer of the prostate, and more than thirty-five thousand will die from this disease each year. Close to one hundred thousand men die of lung cancer each year.

We firmly believe that many of these cancers are preventable. At the end of this chapter, we'll give you specific advice on how melatonin, along with living a healthy lifestyle, can help keep you cancer-free. Before we show how melatonin may be used against cancer, however, we need to explain more about this disease or, to be more accurate, more about these diseases.

CANCER:
THE BREAKDOWN OF IMMUNITY

Many different diseases are lumped under the general heading of cancer, yet they all share one common and deadly thread. Cancer is the uncontrolled growth of abnormal cells that invade and destroy surrounding tissue. We believe that these diseases have something else in common that goes to the root of what cancer really is. We believe that cancer is actually a breakdown in the immune system, or as we called it earlier, the body's surveillance system. In the last chapter, we discussed how the immune system protects the body from unwanted invaders such as viruses or bacteria. We also said that another critical role of the immune system was to attack and eliminate our own cells when they become malignant. Cancer is thus more likely to occur when the immune system slows down, as it does when we age. People with AIDS are notoriously vulnerable to Kaposi's sarcoma and lymphomas despite their age and the rarity of their cancers in the normal population. Since melatonin will slow down the aging of the immune system, we believe that it is a very potent anticancer agent.

Numerous studies—conducted by us and by others—have convinced us that melatonin can boost the immune system, and thus strengthen its ability to root out and destroy cancerous cells. Melatonin increases the aggressiveness and effectiveness of aging T cells, our body's own natural cancer fighters. These are the cells that seek out and destroy abnormal and malignant cells before they can proliferate. As we age, our T cells lose some of their punch, and, not so coincidentally, the rate of cancer climbs in older people. Enhancing the performance of T cells is very important; however, it is only one of the ways that melatonin may protect against cancer.

Cancer can metastasize, or spread, throughout the body via the bloodstream and the lymphatic system. The more it spreads, the more damage it inflicts. We don't know precisely what causes cancer, but there appears to be several factors involved. Cancer is not like a cold that strikes one day and is gone the next; it develops over a long period of time, and occurs in two phases. In the first phase, an initiator begins the process by damaging a cell, causing it to mutate or grow abnormally. As a causative factor, a variety of different conditions can promote the formation of free radicals, unstable oxygen molecules that attack cell membranes and destroy DNA, which is then responsible for initiating the many different types of cancers that afflict us. Many different substances can promote the formation of free radicals, including ultraviolet light, alcohol, radiation, environmental carcinogens such as dioxin, some insecticides, and even viruses. Yet not every mutated cell goes on to become a tumor. In most cases, cells in the immune system knock out these potential troublemakers before they inflict any damage. However, these mutated cells can also lie dormant for years. In the second phase of the cancer process, a promoter or a proliferator encourages these aberrant cells to start dividing.

Many forms of cancer, such as some types of breast cancer and prostate cancer, are called hormone-dependent cancers. If a cancer is hormone-dependent, it means that certain hormones can stimulate it to grow. For example, many studies have shown that when a cell is exposed to estrogen, it alters the cell's normal growth patterns. When a cell's normal growth process is disturbed, it can lead to the growth of tumors. In fact, about two thirds of all breast cancers are estrogen-dependent, which means that exposure to estrogen will promote further growth. Similarly, most prostate cancers are testosterone-dependent, which means that exposure to this male hormone will trigger the growth of the tumor. The precise mechanism by which hormones such as estrogen or testosterone promote cancer is not fully understood. What we do know is that many cells have sites called receptors to which these hormones can bind. When these hormones bind to these receptor sites, it may relay a message to the nucleus of the cell, which stimulates growth. So, for example, if a hormone such as estrogen binds to a dormant cancer cell, it could cause that cell to grow, and the cancer to proliferate. That's why antiestrogens are used to inhibit certain breast cancers.

The Pineal Connection

There is strong evidence that in its role as the regulator of other hormones, melatonin may help prevent hormone-dependent cancers. Some studies have shown that women who have breast cancer often have higher than normal blood levels of estrogen. Studies have also shown a similar link between testosterone in men and prostate cancer. Since melatonin helps the body to maintain normal levels of these hormones, it may very well prevent hormone levels from becoming dangerously high. In fact, we believe, along with many other researchers, that hormone-dependent cancers may indeed be caused by a glitch in the functioning of the pineal gland. Animal studies clearly demonstrate that the removal of the pineal gland can spur the growth and spread of certain types of tumors. Other studies have shown that women with breast cancer and men with prostate cancer both cycle melatonin abnormally, and lack the appropriate nighttime surge of this hormone.

For example, in 1993, at our Third Stromboli Conference on Aging and Cancer, Dr. Christian Bartsch of the University of Tübingen in Germany reported that men with prostate cancer showed many hormonal abnormalities; their thyroid levels were low, their levels of FSH, the hormone that stimulates the production of testosterone, were high, and their levels of prolactin, which stimulates the immune system, were low. What was most striking, however, was the abnormality of melatonin levels that he discerned. Normally, melatonin production peaks at about 2 A.M. and then begins to decline. In men with cancer, however, melatonin production was completely out of whack. Not only were their bodies producing less melatonin than normal, but their melatonin levels increased and decreased at unusual times, peaking in both the afternoon and the night. This was strong evidence that the men's pineal glands, which produce melatonin, were malfunctioning.

As far back as 1978, researchers associated with the National Institutes of Health (NIH) were suggesting that there was a connection between loss of pineal function and disrupted melatonin levels, and breast cancer. In an article that appeared in the distinguished British medical journal *Lancet*, researchers reported that there was a direct statistical correlation between the incidence of breast cancer and the rate of pineal calcification, which can be detected on an X-ray of the skull. In countries with a high rate of pineal calcification, such as the United States, there is a high rate of breast cancer. In countries with a low rate of pineal calcification, such as Japan and Nigeria, there is a low rate of breast cancer. The NIH researchers also reported that melatonin secretion is stimulated by testosterone and estrogen, and that melatonin may "talk back" to the endocrine system to keep those hormones in check. They concluded that the reason young women have a much lower risk of breast cancer than older women is probably due to their higher levels of melatonin.

To further support their case, these researchers cited some interesting data. They reported that psychiatric patients who take the tranquilizer chlorpromazine have a significantly lower rate of breast cancer than the general population. Why? Perhaps, they suggested, it is because chlorpromazine raises melatonin levels. They also noted that early menstruation is a risk factor for developing breast cancer. Why? Perhaps, they suggested, it is because, as other studies have shown, girls having lower melatonin levels are more likely to menstruate earlier than girls with higher melatonin levels. Obese women, they observed, are at greater risk of developing cancer than normal-weight women. Why? Perhaps, they suggested, it is because in obese people melatonin production is disrupted.

A CLOSER LOOK AT MELATONIN

The NIH study spurred other scientists to look more closely at melatonin as an anticancer agent. Several researchers undertook to investigate whether melatonin could impede the growth of breast cancer tumors. In one study, researchers found that blind women, who typically have higher levels of melatonin than normal, have a much lower risk of developing breast cancer. Another study, performed by Steven M. Hill and David E. Blask at the University of Arizona, tested the effect of melatonin on a tissue culture of an estrogen-sensitive human breast cell tumor identified as MCF-7. They found that melatonin did indeed inhibit the growth of these cells by up to 78 percent. Other test tube studies have confirmed that melatonin can inhibit the growth of other kinds of tumor cells as well.

Melatonin not only inhibits the growth of tumor cells in test tubes. It also has been shown to block the growth of breast tumors in laboratory animals, which is significant because cancer grows and spreads in animals the same as it does in humans. In order to assess the effectiveness of a particular substance against cancer, one commonly used technique is to first administer a known carcinogen to an animal, and then administer the potential antidote. In several studies, researchers administered carcinogens known to produce mammary tumors in mice, rats, and hamsters. Then they administered melatonin. In most cases, melatonin either prevented the onset of cancer or significantly slowed its growth.

As we mentioned earlier, prostate cancer is one of the leading causes of death among men over age fifty. The deaths due to prostate cancer of several prominent men in recent years, including Warner Communications CEO Steven Ross, and actors Telly Savalas and Bill Bixby, have called attention to this often lethal disease. As in the case of breast cancer, the growth of prostate tumors may be accelerated by the male hormone testosterone. Although there is no known cure for prostate cancer, it appears as if melatonin can slow down the progression of this disease. In a study conducted at the University of Texas Medical School, researchers found that melatonin could reduce by 50 percent the growth rate of prostatic tumors in rats. If melatonin works as well on human prostatic cancers, it could make a significant difference in the progression of this disease.

Melatonin may thwart the growth of hormone-sensitive tumors by normalizing the production of sex hormones; that, however, is not all it does. Melatonin attacks cancer cells in many different ways. One of the most potent ways to combat cancer is to block the process of cell division, thus nipping the troublesome cells in the bud. When a cell divides, it must undergo a complex sequence of events, one of which is the formation of what scientists call a spindle. Several well-known chemotherapy drugs are what are called spindle poisons. They prevent cells from forming a spindle and thereby prevent them from dividing. These drugs include Taxol, originally derived from the bark of the Pacific yew tree, which is used to treat some types of breast and ovarian cancers, and colchicine-related compounds, which have been used to treat lymphomas. Melatonin also interferes with spindle formation, thereby potentially inhibiting cell division. Thus it may prove to be another important weapon in our chemotherapy arsenal, but one that does not cause the unpleasant side effects that other chemotherapy drugs do.

There's yet another intriguing way in which melatonin may be useful in the treatment of cancer. Studies have shown that melatonin can increase the number of estrogen receptors on human breast cancer cells. Receptors are cells that carry messages from hormones to cells; the hormone gives instructions to the cells via the receptors. Paradoxically, an increase in the number of estrogen receptors on breast cancer cells should promote the growth of breast tumors, and yet, for reasons unknown, in melatonin's case it doesn't. The capacity to increase estrogen receptors, however, can have some genuine therapeutic value. Tamoxifen, one of the most effective and commonly used drugs in the treatment of breast cancer, works by binding with estrogen receptors and inhibiting their effect on cell growth. About 60 percent of all breast tumors are estrogen-sensitive, and many women with these tumors do well on tamoxifen. However, over time, tamoxifen's effectiveness can wear off, and other treatment options are limited. We propose that it may be possible to give these women melatonin to increase their estrogen receptors in order to improve their response to tamoxifen. Indeed, it may also be possible to give melatonin to women who do not have estrogen-sensitive cancers to induce the growth of estrogen receptors so that these women can also respond to tamoxifen. Given the epidemic of breast cancer in the West, these ideas warrant further investigation.

Melatonin may also prevent the initiation of cancer by inhibiting the action of the initiators, the substances that inflict the initial cell damage that causes cells to mutate and become malignant. At the Third Stromboli Conference on Aging and Cancer, noted pineal expert Dr. Russell Reiter reported that melatonin is a highly potent free-radical scavenger. Free radicals are unstable forms of oxygen molecules that can combine at random with components of healthy cells and interfere with normal growth. As we mentioned earlier, healthy cells divide in a methodical fashion. Healthy cells are programmed to know precisely when to stop dividing. When the nucleus of a cell is injured, however, it loses its memory and begins to behave erratically. Cancer occurs when cells begin to grow out of control in a random fashion. The cellular damage inflicted by these free radicals can damage the cell nucleus, and thus promote many different forms of cancer. Free-radical scavengers are molecules that gobble up free radicals before they can do any harm. Dr. Reiter's observations and studies have revealed that melatonin appears to have an affinity for the nucleus of the cell where the DNA is stored. In other words, when melatonin passes through the cell, it finds its way to this important location. This has led some researchers, most notably Dr. Reiter, to speculate that melatonin's specific task may be to protect DNA from the free-radical damage that can cause cancer. Although we find Dr. Reiter's theory to be interesting, we feel that it probably over-states this particular aspect of melatonin. (For more information on how melatonin works as an antioxidant, see Chapter 5.)

Some of the most innovative work on melatonin and cancer is being done outside the United States, in places such as San Gerardo Hospital in Monza, Italy. There, our friend Dr. Paoli Lissoni, one of the most creative researchers in the field of cancer, has conducted some particularly promising studies involving melatonin. We think you should know about them. Lissoni's group has used melatonin alone as a cancer treatment, and in combination with other forms of chemotherapy. In both cases, the results have been very encouraging.

In one study, Lissoni gave only melatonin to patients with a variety of cancers that had already spread from other parts of the body to form inoperable brain tumors. These patients had little hope of recovery. However, those receiving melatonin along with other supportive care fared significantly better than those just receiving supportive care. Specifically, those patients on melatonin lived longer and showed slower tumor progression than the untreated patients. In other studies, Lissoni and his coworkers have combined melatonin with interleukin-2 (IL-2), a natural disease-fighting compound produced by the immune system. In the 1980s, IL-2 was touted as a potential breakthrough in the treatment of certain types of cancers, and it is approved by the FDA for the treatment of renal cancer in the United States. However, the side effects of IL-2 are nothing short of terrible. This drug, which is quite toxic, can produce high fevers, chills, water retention, swelling, and other problems. IL-2 may do a good job of wiping out cancer cells, but few patients can tolerate its side effects. Lissoni, however, devised an ingenious approach. He used a lower and less toxic dose of IL-2 and combined it with melatonin. He administered IL-2 and melatonin to patients with a wide variety of cancers, including kidney, stomach, and liver cancer and even melanoma. Once again, these were patients who had little hope of long-term survival. After the IL-2/melatonin program, many of these patients showed marked improvement —their tumors regressed, their appetites returned, and they seemed to be generally doing better. A handful of patients even appeared to experience partial remissions. Moreover, the melatonin was able to virtually eliminate the severe side effects of IL-2, making the immunotherapy treatment far more tolerable. Follow-up studies have showed that although the IL-2/melatonin regimen did not result in any miracle cures, it did appear to extend the lives of many patients, and perhaps, more importantly, to improve the quality of their lives.

One of Lissoni's most interesting studies established a link between melatonin levels and patient response to cancer therapy. In his study of forty-two chemotherapy patients, Lissoni tested their melatonin levels before chemotherapy and also four weeks after the end of their treatment. Lissoni found a direct correlation between patient improvement and a rise in melatonin levels. Out of the sixteen patients who had shown a rise in melatonin levels, tumors shrank in twelve and did not progress in the rest. Out of the twenty-six patients who had shown a continuous fall in melatonin, only two showed any improvement. Melatonin levels may indeed be a marker that can help doctors predict the prognosis of their cancer patients.

In addition to Lissoni's work, there are other examples of how melatonin may enhance the effect of traditional chemotherapy, while sparing patients some of its horrendous side effects. Under the direction of Dr. Bruno Neri, researchers at the University of Florence in Italy tested the effect of melatonin combined with another anticancer drug, human lymphoblastoid interferon (HLI). HLI is a natural protein that can kill viruses and cancer cells, but also causes miserable side effects, including fever, chills, and muscle aches. In Neri's study, twenty-one patients with progressive renal cell carcinoma—a particularly insidious form of kidney cancer that can spread quickly, and is often unresponsive to chemotherapy—were given HLI and melatonin. In past studies, HLI had been shown to be only mildly effective against this cancer. When combined with melatonin, however, the HLI appeared to work better, and the side effects were lessened. In fact, in three patients the tumors disappeared completely, although only follow-up studies will show if this is a true and lasting cure. Four patients showed partial remissions. As of this writing, Neri is conducting a larger study to determine if HLI and melatonin will prove to be an effective treatment for this potentially deadly form of cancer.

The studies that we've just described show that melatonin, when combined with traditional chemotherapy, not only can improve the performance of anticancer drugs, but can also lessen the severity of side effects, and actually makes the patients feel better. This makes perfect sense given what we know about melatonin. Our studies have shown that melatonin works in combination with the natural opiates or painkillers produced in our bodies. When we're sick and under a great deal of stress, or in pain due to an injury, our bodies produce chemical compounds called endorphins, which help relieve pain. The immune system is instrumental in the release of certain endorphins, and in fact, these hormones may also play a role in healing. Such studies suggest that melatonin may work in tandem with these natural opiates, and may enhance their action. Perhaps this is why the cancer patients felt better when taking melatonin. In fact, it's also possible that when melatonin is combined with other narcotics or tranquilizers, there might be a synergistic effect, that is, the two combined may be stronger than the effect of any one alone. In this respect, melatonin may be beneficial for cancer patients, or any patients suffering pain, since it decreases the need for narcotics and minimizes negative side effects.

One of the problems with many of the most effective forms of chemotherapy is that the cure is almost as bad as the disease itself in terms of the harm it can inflict on the body. By necessity, chemotherapy drugs must be strong enough to knock out cancer cells, and very often they also destroy healthy cells in the process. For example, some anticancer drugs can destroy the blood-forming cells in the bone marrow, which can result in severe anemia, and can inflict untold damage on the immune system. We investigated whether melatonin might actually protect the bone marrow from this kind of damage. With Vladimir Lesnikov in St. Petersburg, we tested the toxicity of several chemotherapy agents on the bone marrow cells of mice. We put the cells in a test tube and mixed them with different anticancer drugs. Our results confirmed that when melatonin was added to the brew, the bone marrow cells suffered far less damage. This is yet another aspect of melatonin that is worthy of further investigation.

Our findings are consistent with those of other researchers who have shown that chemotherapy is often more effective and less toxic when given at night, presumably because melatonin levels are at their peak. In fact, many chemotherapy patients are now given intravenous pumps with timers that automatically pulse anticancer drugs into their bodies while they sleep. Thanks to this innovation, many of these patients are now able to get their chemotherapy treatments in the comfort of their own home, which is a much more natural and relaxing setting than a hospital. This also means that the treatment does not disrupt normal sleep patterns—and nighttime melatonin production—which can be disturbed by the bright lights and noise of a busy hospital.

MELATONIN AND EMFS

Over the past century, the incidence of certain forms of cancer, notably breast cancer, prostate cancer, and certain types of leukemia, has risen dramatically throughout the developed world. What has triggered the higher incidence of these cancers? Is it a result of diet, lifestyle, or environmental pollution? With these questions in mind, pathologists at the University of Toronto Sunnybrook Health Science Center reviewed all the possible factors that may have contributed to the rise in cancer. They examined the effects of air pollution, smoking, occupational hazards, stress, and other suspected carcinogens. They concluded that there has been one important change over the past century that may have done more to contribute to the rise in cancer than any other factor. During this period, we went from a society that was dependent on candlelight to one that is dependent on electric light. Numerous studies have shown that exposure to artificial light can suppress the production of melatonin, which, as we have just seen, is an anticancer agent. These researchers concluded that because artificial light can inhibit melatonin production, the proliferation of electric lighting may be the primary cause of the increase in cancer. End of story.

Not so fast, say other researchers, who believe that this explanation is at best only half the story. They point out that the spread of electric lights was not an isolated event; it was due to the spread of electric power, and that also has been cited as a potential cancer-causing agent. Indeed, some highly respected scientists contend that the spread of electric power is the main reason cancer rates are on the rise. But the mere mention of the words "electricity" and "cancer" in tandem will trigger hot debate in the research community.

You may be wondering what electricity has to do with cancer. Electricity emits invisible forces called electromagnetic fields or EMFs for short. There is some evidence that EMFs may interfere with the evening production of melatonin, and that is why some researchers believe that exposure to EMFs may also be a possible cause of many different types of cancers.

If this is correct, it is worrisome indeed. EMFs are everywhere. They radiate from overhead power lines, computers, fax machines, and portable telephones. In fact, the earth itself radiates electromagnetic waves that are actually much higher than the waves emitted by power lines. In your home, EMFs are emitted by refrigerators, hair dryers, electric shavers, electric blankets, computers, and other appliances. There is no escaping them—they can pass from one room to another through the walls. There's no debating the fact that EMFs are everywhere; the question is, do these invisible rays pose a significant threat?

Earlier studies have suggested that there may be an increase in cancer among children who live near high-current power lines. Naturally, these studies have frightened people, and have encouraged a movement in the United States and abroad to force electric companies to either install protective shielding around their power lines or to put them underground, which is a very expensive proposition and not likely to be done in the near future.

The National Cancer Institute is now investigating whether EMFs pose a significant health risk, but it will be several years before we know for sure. So far, the studies on EMFs have been confusing and inconclusive. Recently, the American Physical Society, the members of which include some of the nation's top physicists, announced that the public's fear of overhead power lines was completely groundless. The group based its conclusion on a review of more than one thousand studies. It took the position that concern over power lines was diverting attention from more important environmental issues.

Nevertheless, some studies have suggested a link between certain occupations known for high EMF exposure—such as telephone and electric line workers—and certain types of cancers. Curiously, men—but not necessarily women—who work in these occupations appear to have a higher risk of breast cancer. In fact, one study did show that men in electrical occupations had six times the risk of breast cancer than normal. But in keeping with the general inconsistencies of studies in this field, many other studies have found no link between male electrical workers and breast cancer. It's been even more difficult to document the connection between EMFs and breast cancer in women.

One recent study did find such a link, but it has generated so much controversy that even its own authors question what it really shows. Researchers at the University of North Carolina studied U.S. death records for 1985 to 1989. The researchers isolated the records of women who worked in electrical occupations, and compared their rate of death due to breast cancer to a control group of women who did not work in these high-risk occupations. The study showed that the women in electrical occupations had a 38 percent greater risk of dying from breast cancer than did other working women. But there were many inconsistencies in the study that confounded the researchers. For example, although electrical engineers and telephone installers had a much higher risk of dying from breast cancer than normal, telephone or computer operators did not show any increased risk. What is curious about this finding is that an electrical engineer is usually a white-collar, supervisory job, where the exposure to EMFs would presumably be much lower than among the blue-collar workers. If anything, electrical engineers spend their days in front of a computer terminal, and yet computer operators showed no increased risk. One of the problems with this study is that the subjects were all dead and could not be questioned further. The researchers had to take it on faith that the women described their occupation accurately. There was also no way of knowing other potentially significant factors such as the presence of power lines near a workplace, and the true level of EMF exposure on the job. No one questioned the accuracy or integrity of these researchers; by all accounts, they did the best with what data they had. Although this study may have actually generated more questions than it answered, many scientists are unwilling to dismiss the possibility that EMFs may indeed be a causal factor in cancer.

Some, but not all, in vitro studies of human breast cancer cells show that EMFs may trigger the growth of cancerous cells by blocking the anticancer action of melatonin. In one study conducted at the University of California at Berkeley, researchers exposed human estrogen-dependent breast cancer cells and melatonin to a sixty-hertz magnetic field, the kind of low-frequency EMFs emitted by power lines and common appliances. The study showed that the EMFs prevented melatonin from inhibiting the growth of these cells. How significant is this finding? Does it necessarily mean that EMFs could be causing human breast cancer cells to grow by inhibiting melatonin? No one knows. What's even more confusing is that some animal studies found that low-level exposure to EMFs did not seem to promote the growth of breast tumors.

A growing number of researchers believe that only some kinds of EMFs are dangerous. For example, Russell Reiter has proposed that only EMFs characterized by rapid pulses and quick changes in the magnetic field—such as those emitted by a handheld hair dryer or an electric blanket—are dangerous, but this has not yet been proven.

In fact, a recent study published in *Nature* raises some important questions about studies that had been conducted on the relationship between EMFs and cancer. Researchers at Oregon State University proposed that the past studies on EMFs could be seriously flawed because the scientists performing them failed to consider the effect of microscopic magnets (called crystals of magnetite) in the environment, which could interact with the EMFs used in the studies. These microscopic magnets are everywhere—in our air, in water, and, according to the *Nature* article, on the commercially prepared medium used to grow cell cultures, and even in plastic labware. In fact, the Oregon State researchers simulated an EMF culture trial, but omitted one important thing—the live cells. They found that the culture had become so contaminated with these micromagnets that it would have been impossible to conduct an accurate study demonstrating the effect of EMFs. The Oregon State group proposed that EMFs may be harmful, but for a different reason than had been originally suspected. They suggested that these tiny crystals of magnetite, recently discovered to be plentiful in the brain and other human tissue, may interact with EMFs in a harmful way.

Given the contradictory information on EMFs, what precautions, if any, should people take? Indeed, some people are so concerned about this potential threat that they are buying special devices to measure EMFs in their homes and are frantically replacing appliances and rearranging furniture. We're not convinced that the threat is a real one, yet we're not ready to dismiss it entirely either. If you are truly concerned about EMFs, we recommend a more conservative—and we believe sensible—approach. We live in an industrialized society and short of moving to a remote island, no one is going to be able to completely avoid exposure to EMFs. We don't think it's necessary to give up your refrigerator or even your hair dryer. However, there are some potentially harmful situations that can easily be avoided without going to extremes. For example, if you use a computer, make sure that you're using it safely. We know that the strongest electrical fields are emitted from the sides and back of a computer screen. Therefore, if you work on a computer, try to sit at least an arm's length away. If you work in a room with several computers, move your chair away from the back or sides of others' computers. We're not even going to advise you to throw out your electric blanket, but if you must use one, stick to one of the newer-model blankets that have a significantly lower output of EMFs. Perhaps supplementing and maintaining our nighttime melatonin levels can provide the solution to all our concerns regarding EMFs.

Frankly, when it comes to EMFs, we're still in the dark about what if any threat they may pose. Until we know more about EMFs and cancer, simple steps to avoid overexposure probably make sense, but going to extremes to avoid EMFs is to us nonsensical.

TIPS ON CANCER PREVENTION

In this chapter, we've shown how melatonin shows promise as a powerful cancer fighter and how it is already being used to treat different forms of this disease.

If so much talk about cancer has left you with the

impression that getting the disease is inevitable, let us close this chapter by stating emphatically that it most certainly is not. Cancer is very much a preventable disease. This is not just our opinion, it is an accepted fact. According to the National Cancer Institute, perhaps as many as half of all cancers can be avoided by making simple changes in lifestyle and diet. For example, by not smoking cigarettes you can significantly reduce the odds of getting cancer. By eating a diet rich in fruits and vegetables you can further tip the scales in your favor. Fruits and vegetables contain fiber and many other important compounds called phytochemicals that have been shown to fight cancer in many different ways, and at different stages of the disease. Needless to say, we both eat large quantities of these foods and try to live a healthy lifestyle. But most importantly, we both take melatonin. Melatonin combats cancer on many different fronts in many different ways. It strengthens your immune system's ability to spot and destroy abnormal cells that may turn cancerous, and it prevents the age-related decline in immunity that leaves you vulnerable to cancer. It can thwart the growth and spread of cancerous tumors. It can dampen the effect of hormones that can trigger the growth of certain types of cancers, including breast cancer and prostate cancer. Melatonin is a multifaceted anticancer compound that may help to keep us cancer-free.

If you already have cancer, we also believe that a relatively low dose of melatonin (5 to 10 mg) daily during your course of treatment could be very beneficial. If you have cancer, and are interested in taking melatonin along with your conventional therapy, we urge you to talk to your doctor or oncologist before self-medicating. We are both physicians, and we feel very strongly that a patient and a doctor should work together. If your physician is unaware of melatonin's role in cancer therapy, he or she can learn more about it by reading some of the articles cited in the extensive bibliography that appears at the end of this book. As we mentioned earlier, melatonin can enhance the effect of painkillers and tranquilizers, and if you are on any of these types of medications, you may need to reduce your dose if you take melatonin.

CHAPTER 8

Melatonin:
For a Strong Heart

THE PROMISE OF MELATONIN:
- Normalizes blood cholesterol levels
- Lowers high blood pressure
- Protects body from stress-induced illness
- Helps to prevent heart attack and stroke

Although they have markedly different functions, the pineal gland and the heart share some striking similarities. Both are powerhouses within the body. The pineal gland must continuously regulate, monitor, and superintend every other gland and organ in the body. The heart is equally energetic. It beats a hundred thousand times each day, pumping blood with its life-sustaining oxygen and nutrients to every cell in the body. The heart beats two and a half billion times during the course of an average life span. It nourishes the glands and organs that the pineal controls.

In light of the incredibly important roles that the heart and the pineal gland play in sustaining life, the fact that philosophers throughout the ages have attributed mystical powers to both of these organs is not at all surprising. The Greek philosopher Aristotle believed that the soul actually resided in the heart. The ancient Egyptians believed that the fate of the soul was determined by the weight of the heart. The French philosopher Descartes thought the soul operated through the pineal. Hindu mystics believed that the soul departed from the body after death through the pineal.

These philosophers had keen intuition. The pineal and the heart are inextricably linked in subtle but important ways. In fact, the pineal—which we have come to think of as the "heart of the brain"—helps to keep the "heart of the body" strong and resilient, and functioning well throughout our lives. It does this through its hormone, melatonin, which transmits its messages throughout the body.

When the heart stops pumping, the results are disastrous: The blood stops circulating throughout the body, and within half an hour the cells in the vital organs, including the heart itself, suffocate and die. In the Western world, heart disease is the number one killer of both men and women; it accounts for half of all deaths that occur annually. As we age, and our levels of melatonin begin to decline, we become particularly vulnerable to heart disease. Fortunately, there are ways to prevent heart disease, and melatonin can be a useful tool in keeping you "strong at heart."

In this chapter, we will explain the different ways that melatonin helps preserve and protect the heart. If you don't have heart disease, you may be tempted to skip over this chapter. This could be the mistake of your life. Many of the problems we are addressing in this chapter are symptomless or have symptoms that are very subtle. You may suffer from one or more of these problems without the slightest awareness of it. Surprisingly, many of these problems are striking people—especially women—at younger and younger ages. Therefore, we recommend that you review the material in this chapter so that you are at least aware of these conditions, if only to take the necessary steps to prevent them.

MELATONIN: REGULATOR OF CHOLESTEROL

Most deaths due to heart disease are actually caused by coronary artery disease or CAD. Think of an artery as a garden hose; blood flows through the hose to get to the heart. CAD occurs when the arteries supplying blood to the heart become clogged with plaque, a thick, yellowish, waxy substance that restricts the flow of blood through the arteries. When an artery becomes clogged, the condition is called atherosclerosis. Plaque contains many different types of cells, including cholesterol, a fat or lipid produced by the liver and other specialized cells throughout the body. Plaque deposits can build up over time. Eventually, they can grow to the point that they block the flow of blood to the heart. Although scientists have come up with many plausible theories, exactly why these arteries fill up with plaque is still unclear. We do know the devastating result of plaque formation, however: When the blood cannot get to the heart muscle, the heart cells are deprived of oxygen, and portions of the heart may be permanently damaged. This is what happens when someone has a heart attack.

Although cholesterol appears to be the primary culprit in plaque formation, cholesterol, in and of itself, is not dangerous. Indeed, the body could not live without it. Cholesterol performs many important functions. It is essential for the production of sex hormones, it is needed to produce myelin, the fatty sheath that insulates nerves, and it is required for the synthesis of vitamin D. Too much cholesterol, however, can cause serious problems.

Cholesterol is not only produced by the body, but is found in many foods such as eggs, meat, and others derived from animal products. Cholesterol is also produced from saturated fat, which is also abundant in meat and dairy products. A small percentage of people have a genetic defect that causes their cells to pump out too much cholesterol; this is called familial hypercholesterolemia. However, studies suggest that many people who have high cholesterol tend to eat diets high in fat, and, in fact, reducing your fat intake can help cut cholesterol. In addition, there are some drugs that can keep cholesterol levels within normal levels.

"Normal" is the operative word when it comes to cholesterol. Studies have shown that people who have very low cholesterol levels have a higher incidence of cancer, and what's even more surprising, a higher rate of suicide. No one knows the relationship between cholesterol and cancer, but some researchers suspect that the disease itself may cause a drop in cholesterol levels. Why there is a correlation between very low cholesterol and suicide is a complete mystery. In the United States normal cholesterol is defined as 120 to 220 mg/dl per deciliter of blood. Anything over 200 mg/dl may increase your risk of developing heart disease, but there are other variables that affect the incidence of disease. Even more significant is the ratio between two types of cholesterol, HDL (high-density lipoprotein) and LDL (low-density lipoprotein). In recent years, HDL has become known as the "good" cholesterol, because it carries cholesterol to the liver for secretion in the bile. In other words, it rids excess cholesterol from your body. On the other hand, LDL has become known as the "bad" cholesterol because it carries cholesterol throughout the bloodstream. Ideally, the ratio between total cholesterol and HDL should not exceed 6:1.

Triglyceride is another blood lipid that needs to be monitored, especially by women. In fact, in women in particular, high triglyceride levels (defined as anything over 190 mg/dl) greatly increases their risk of having a heart attack. (For men, triglycerides over 400 mg/dl are considered dangerous.)

The pineal gland appears to play a major role in normalizing cholesterol and other important blood lipids. When the pineal gland was removed in animals, both their cholesterol and triglyceride levels soared. Other animal studies have verified melatonin's positive effect on blood lipids. For example, in one study performed at the University of Tokyo, researchers designed an experiment to determine if melatonin could lower cholesterol in rats. There were four groups of rats in the study. One group was fed a normal diet and a melatonin supplement, and a control group was fed a normal diet without the melatonin. A second group of rats was given a high-cholesterol diet and a melatonin supplement, and the control group was fed a high-cholesterol diet without the melatonin.

The melatonin had little discernible effect on the rats that were fed a normal diet. However, the effect of melatonin on the rats who were fed a high-cholesterol diet was nothing short of remarkable. Melatonin appeared to blunt the effect of cholesterol intake on blood levels of cholesterol. Although the rats who were fed a high-cholesterol diet and melatonin did experience some rise in cholesterol levels, the increase was far less than that for the control group, the rats who were fed a high-cholesterol diet without any melatonin supplement. This is a prime example of how melatonin operates as a "smart" hormone. It is selective in its action: It works only when and where it is needed, and does not attempt to fix something that is not broken. In this experiment, the melatonin did not try to lower cholesterol in rats that were fed a normal diet; it only went to work in rats that were fed the high-cholesterol diet.

We believe that melatonin will help normalize cholesterol levels in those of us whose cholesterol levels are too high. We have recommended melatonin for this purpose, and there is anecdotal evidence that it works. A case in point is a friend of Walter's who had undergone quadruple bypass surgery to treat atherosclerosis. When coronary arteries become so clogged that blood can no longer pass through them and feed the heart, an artery is taken from another part of the body, such as the leg, and attached to the heart and to a point on the clogged artery downstream from the obstruction. Thus the blood is detoured, or bypassed around the blockage. After the bypass surgery, Walter's friend was not doing well. His blood lipid and sugar levels remained dangerously high, he had grown frail and tired, and he was having difficulty sleeping. When Walter heard him describe these symptoms, he recommended that his friend take 5 mg of melatonin at night. When Walter met up with his friend months later, the change was startling. The friend looked stronger and healthier (which he attributed to a new-found ability to sleep soundly), and, much to his physician's amazement, his blood lipid and sugar levels had normalized. His metabolism is now being kept permanently balanced with melatonin. We believe that melatonin made the difference.

How does melatonin lower high cholesterol? We do not know for certain, but we believe it has to do with the effect melatonin has on the thyroid gland's production of hormones. As discussed earlier, the thyroid gland is a butterfly-shaped gland located at the base of the neck. The thyroid gland produces two hormones, T_4 and T_3, which are both involved in cell metabolism, that is, the process by which the cells utilize energy. T_4 and T_3 are instrumental in the breakdown and utilization of cholesterol in the body. In fact, people with underactive thyroid glands, a condition called hypothyroidism, typically have high blood cholesterol levels, which are normalized when they are given thyroid hormone-replacement therapy. Melatonin controls the breakdown of thyroid hormones from T_4 to T_3. T_3 is the more powerful of the two thyroid hormones and it burns energy faster. T_3 breaks cholesterol down and utilizes it faster. We believe that by increasing the level of T_3 hormone, melatonin increases the rate at which cholesterol is broken down in the body and utilized.

CONTROLLING BLOOD PRESSURE

Hypertension, or high blood pressure, is one of the most insidious of all diseases. Called the silent killer because it is painless and often symptomless, high blood pressure is a leading risk factor for heart attack, stroke, loss of vision, and kidney disease.

Blood pressure measures the force exerted by blood on the arterial wall (the hose carrying blood from the heart). Normal blood pressure is defined at about 120/80. The top number measures the systolic pressure, the pressure in the artery at the moment when the heart contracts and pushes blood into the arteries. The bottom number measures the diastolic pressure, the pressure in the arteries when the heart muscle relaxes between beats. As we age, our blood pressure tends to rise, in many cases to unhealthy levels. A blood pressure reading above 140/90 is considered to be high blood pressure. About sixty million Americans have high blood pressure and it is a particular problem among African-Americans. Many physicians believe that even a slight increase in pressure can substantially increase the risk of heart or kidney disease.

There is strong evidence that melatonin protects against high blood pressure. Interestingly, when we sleep, and we are pumping out melatonin, our heart rate slows down and our blood pressure drops. However, when our melatonin levels drop by early morning, there is a sharp rise in blood pressure. You may be surprised to know that the hours of 6 A.M. to 9 A.M. are known as the "witching hours" in cardiac-care units, because these are the hours during which most heart attacks occur. To us, this is not surprising. We know that when the pineal gland is removed from animals, their melatonin levels drop, and as a result, they experience an immediate and permanent rise in blood pressure.

There are other tantalizing clues that melatonin is an important regulator of blood pressure. When melatonin cycles through the bloodstream, it passes through the kidneys. The kidneys play an important role in governing blood pressure. The kidney secretes several hormones, including aldosterone and renin, which control salt retention, blood volume, and other factors that can influence blood pressure. (This is why people with high blood pressure or heart failure are often told to take diuretics or water pills, which rid the body of excess fluid.) We believe that in the kidneys, melatonin functions as a sort of buffer hormone that normalizes the levels of other kidney hormones, and thus keeps blood pressure levels in check.

Controlling "Killer" Stress

Living under constant stress can have a devastating effect on both the hearts and souls of men and women. Although it may take longer to do its destructive work, chronic, nagging stress can be as lethal as a bullet to the heart. When we are under stress, the brain signals to the body to react in a specific way. The sympathetic (also known as autonomic) nervous system takes over and the body gets fired up for action. The adrenal glands secret the hormones epinephrine (also called adrenaline) and norepinephrine, which cause the heart to race. Our blood pressure rises. The pupils in our eyes dilate, allowing more light to enter for better night vision, and the body burns more oxygen to fuel these changes. We also begin to pump corticosteroid and other hormones. We call this the flight or fight response.

All of this takes its toll on the heart and brain. Studies have shown that even in the absence of arterial disease, the heart is vulnerable to stress-related injury. In fact, one very dramatic study in rats showed that stress alone could induce severe damage to the heart muscle, not unlike the kind of damage that results from a heart attack. Certain steroids produced under stress, such as corticosteroids, have been shown to be particularly damaging to the heart. Similarly, stress steroids can damage the hippocampus, a part of the brain involved in the storage and transfer of memory. Melatonin can protect against the devastating effects of stress in a very important way. Melatonin decreases the production of corticosteroids and thus can help dampen their lethal effect on the heart. (For more information on stress, see Chapter 11.)

THE MITOCHONDRIA CONNECTION

When the pineal gland grows old, it develops calcium deposits, as do other organs in the body, including, notably, the heart. Calcium deposits can make an organ stiff and slow to react. If calcium deposits grow in the blood vessels that carry blood to the heart, they can block the flow of blood to the heart, and cause a heart attack. Calcification can also occur in the heart muscle itself, and this can interfere with the heart's ability to pump blood.

No one knows precisely what causes the heart or blood vessels to calcify, but we speculate that, like the aging process itself, the process is yet another result of a decline in the functioning of the pineal gland. The pineal gland is one of the most active glands in the body, and it utilizes a great deal of energy. It gets energy from mitochondria, the tiny structure within each cell of the body that are known as the powerhouse of the cell. Mitochondria produce ATP (adenosine triphosphate), the fuel that enables the body to maintain its heat and to keep running. ATP is what provides the cells in the pineal with the energy to produce melatonin, and the cells in the heart with the energy to keep beating. As the pineal ages, its mitochondria produce less ATP, and more of another compound called pyrophosphate. Pyrophosphate binds with calcium and forms calcium salt deposits within the pineal. Once it begins to calcify, the pineal begins to run down, and it produces less melatonin. If you remember, we said earlier that melatonin helps to break down thyroid hormone to its most potent, energy-producing form. The cells need this energy so that they can continue to make more ATP or fuel. Without enough energy to carry on the production of ATP, cells in other organs such as the heart would begin to produce excess pyrophosphate, which in turn binds with calcium to form the calcium salt deposits that have become the hallmark of aging.

How can we break this destructive cycle? We believe that melatonin-replacement therapy may help keep the pineal-producing ATP at youthful levels, localize and protect mitochondria throughout the body, and as a result can prevent this entire cascade of events from occurring.

ANTIOXIDANTS AND THE HEART

Although we are all too familiar with the devastating effects of heart disease, its precise cause is still unknown, although many interesting theories have been offered. Some experts feel that diet plays a major role. They believe that a high-fat diet can trigger the production of excess cholesterol, which winds up as artery-clogging plaque. It has been very hard, however, for science to prove this thesis. Although studies have confirmed the link between high cholesterol levels and heart disease, none have actually proved that eating a high-fat diet will lead to high cholesterol levels.

Recently, the role of antioxidants in preventing heart disease has been a subject of great interest to the medical community and the public at large. Many researchers believe that the plaque that blocks the blood flow begins to grow in the artery as a result of an injury to the inner core of the artery. What causes this injury? Researchers speculate that the initial injury may be caused by the oxidation of LDL, or "bad" cholesterol, by free radicals, or unstable oxygen molecules. Once oxidized or injured, the LDL cholesterol may attract scavenger cells that gobble it up and form something called foam cells, which begin the formation of plaque. If this theory is correct, then substances called free-radical scavengers can prevent the initial injury from occurring by gobbling up the free radicals before they can attack the LDL.

Melatonin is a free-radical scavenger, which, according to our studies, and the work of others, works at least as well as vitamin E in protecting against the harm inflicted by free radicals in the bloodstream. If melatonin works as well as vitamin E in preventing heart disease, it is doing a good job indeed. In one major study of forty thousand male health professionals, those taking a vitamin E supplement had a 40 percent reduced risk of developing heart disease. Based on these studies and similar ones, we believe that melatonin can have the same positive effect.

Melatonin is an extremely useful tool in helping to prevent heart disease, the number one killer of both men and women. Its heart-healthy effects are felt in several ways. Melatonin can lower cholesterol, thereby preventing the formation of plaque deposits that can clog arteries and block the flow of blood. Melatonin can normalize blood pressure, and inhibit the action of free radicals, both of which can destroy arteries and injure the heart. Melatonin can even blunt the destructive effects of corticosteroids, stress hormones that can inflict damage to heart muscle in an otherwise healthy body.

In sum, melatonin will help to keep our hearts strong and efficient for our entire lives.

CHAPTER 9

Exciting Frontiers:
The Promise of the Future

When we decided to write this book, one of our goals was to alert both the public and the scientific community to the role of melatonin in treating many illnesses, and thereby encourage further serious research in this area. Based on what we already know about melatonin, we think that when such research is undertaken it will demonstrate that this amazing hormone can be used to treat, and prevent, quite a number of diseases.

In this chapter we will explore what we believe are some of melatonin's potential medical applications for the future, which include the treatment of AIDS, Alzheimer's disease, and blindness.

As you read this chapter and learn more about melatonin and its disease-fighting potential, we are sure that you will agree that melatonin has great promise indeed as a disease-fighting hormone and that more research must be done.

ACQUIRED IMMUNE DEFICIENCY SYNDROME (AIDS)

AIDS—acquired immune deficiency syndrome—is not one disease, but a group of diseases that result from the suppression of the immune system by a retrovirus, a virus that can alter the genetic makeup of a cell. That retrovirus is known as the human immunodeficiency virus or HIV. HIV is a slow-acting virus; it is possible to test positive for HIV antibodies—which means that one has been exposed to the virus—without actually having AIDS. AIDS is defined as the presence of two or more related illnesses in persons who have tested positive for HIV. There is some debate in the scientific community as to whether everyone who tests positive for HIV will necessarily develop AIDS. Most researchers believe that people who are HIV positive will eventually develop AIDS, although it may be years before they do. To us, AIDS represents a microcosm of the aging process itself, because it involves the weakening and destruction of the immune system and a resulting wasting syndrome that epitomizes senescence. Looking at advanced AIDS patients, we find ourselves thinking that they look old beyond their years.

When AIDS was first recognized in the United States in 1979, it was found primarily in the male homosexual community, but it did not stay confined to that population. Today, there are more than ten million people worldwide who are infected with HIV, and, in the United States, it is spreading the fastest among women and teenagers.

It is now generally well understood that HIV can be transmitted through semen, blood and blood products, and breast milk. Unlike some highly contagious diseases such as tuberculosis, the AIDS virus cannot be passed through the air or through coughing or sneezing, or through casual contact, such as shaking hands. In fact, if you take proper precautions, AIDS can be prevented. Since there is no cure and few effective treatments, prevention is truly the best medicine.

Although we have not been able to identify any studies of the use of melatonin as a treatment for AIDS, based on what we do know about the immune system, and the role melatonin plays in strengthening it, we believe that melatonin may also play a useful role in helping to slow down the progression of this disease. We recommend more research in this area.

What makes HIV so insidious and difficult to control is the way it specifically targets and attacks the immune system. In particular, HIV decimates two types of T cells or lymphocytes, called CD-4 and CD-8. Both of these cells play a critical role in keeping the immune system functioning. CD-4 cells protect other cells from foreign proteins, viruses, and other trespassing organisms. CD-8 cells produce antibodies that circulate through the bloodstream seeking out and destroying potential troublemakers. People with HIV have much lower levels of these important T cells. As a result, they are more prone to so-called opportunistic infections. These are infections that prey on weakened immune systems. For example, people with AIDS are especially vulnerable to Pneumocystis carinii pneumonia (PCP) and cytomegalovirus (CMV), which causes blindness. When a person with a healthy immune system encounters the organisms that cause these infections, he or she is usually able to fight them off. Fending them off is not so easy for persons with compromised immune systems. For them, even a relatively minor infection can develop into a life-threatening disease. Researchers have developed several treatments that appear to help prevent some of these opportunistic infections from taking hold, and

HIV-infected people should know of them in discussions of treatments with their doctors.

We believe that melatonin, since it helps strengthen the immune system, may also help HIV-compromised immune systems fight off infections. Moreover, as a hormone that has been shown to stimulate the immune system, we think that melatonin may help preserve immune function and slow down the progression from HIV to AIDS. We base our opinion on our earlier work on the immune system, which has demonstrated that melatonin can have a positive effect on the production of T cells.

You will recall from earlier chapters, for example, that some of our research on melatonin and immunity involved what are called athymic nude mice. These are mice born without a thymus gland. The thymus gland, which is located in the chest, is an important component of the immune system. The thymus gland is where our T cells are stored until they are called upon to fight infections. In many ways, these athymic nude mice are similar to AIDS patients. Both have weakened immunity, and both are subject to dying at an early age as a result of infection. However, we were able to restore T cell production by increasing melatonin levels in these mice. We did this in two ways. In one series of experiments, we transplanted a pineal gland from normal mice into the athymic nude mice and thereby increased their melatonin production. In another series of experiments, we added melatonin to the nighttime drinking water of the athymic nude mice. In both experiments, the melatonin-treated or pineal-transplanted mice stayed healthier, and lived significantly longer, than their untreated counterparts. Thus we believe that melatonin can play an important role in strengthening the immune systems of people with AIDS.

We have noted before that the process of aging exacts a toll on the immune system similar to the damage the HIV virus inflicts. Like people with AIDS, older people typically have a diminished immune response. Their T cells are not nearly as aggressive as they were when they were younger. That is why the elderly are so vulnerable to infections that younger people can shake off. Aging animals have the same immune deficiency problems as aging people. Therefore it bears repeating that our experiments demonstrated that melatonin significantly boosted the immune systems of older mice, and raised their T cell production to levels typical of younger mice.

Melatonin may also help control the stress that is associated with a chronic illness such as AIDS. People with AIDS typically have a high output of corticosteroids. Corticosteroids are known as stress hormones because they are released by the adrenal glands during times of stress, such as when we are angry, upset, feel threatened, or are sick. Corticosteroids reduce inflammation caused by infections, but in so doing they also dampen the immune system by blocking the action of disease-fighting T cells. This effect is, of course, precisely the opposite of what an AIDS patient needs. Melatonin helps to control corticosteroid production, and as a result may reduce the effect of corticosteroids on our immune systems.

There is yet another important way that melatonin may help in the fight against AIDS, and that is by protecting glutathione, an antioxidant that is produced by immune cells. Antioxidants such as glutathione protect our bodies against oxidative damage inflicted by free radicals, the unstable molecules that can injure cells and cause them to mutate. Free radicals can also inflict damage on naturally occurring antioxidants, such as glutathione. Melatonin can help protect glutathione from free-radical damage, according to a recent study, and thus enhance the ability of glutathione to protect other cells. The significance of this, insofar as people with AIDS are concerned, is that, as we explained above, AIDS patients have low T cell levels. There is evidence that this occurs because T cells are destroyed by damage inflicted by free radicals due to a depletion of the protective antioxidant glutathione. If melatonin can protect glutathione, then glutathione can, in turn, continue to protect against the destruction of these critical T cells.

The human immune system is extremely complex, and AIDS is a very clever and deadly disease. We are not suggesting that melatonin can cure AIDS, and we certainly don't want to raise false hopes. We do believe, however, that melatonin is safe and may give the immune system a much needed boost that may help sustain life until new and better treatments can be found. For people who are HIV positive, we recommend a dose of melatonin of 5 to 10 mg each evening. We discuss how to take melatonin in more detail in Chapter 14 of this book.

In addition to taking melatonin, HIV positive people should take other steps to maintain a strong immune system. Getting enough rest, eating well, and avoiding excess stress are especially important to strengthening immunity.

ALZHEIMER'S DISEASE

Of all the diseases associated with aging, Alzheimer's disease is the one that is most dreaded and feared, and with good reason. It is an absolutely devastating disease that diminishes every aspect of life. Alzheimer's disease is characterized by the irreversible loss of memory, rational thought, and ability to communicate. As the disease progresses, its victims lose awareness of themselves and their environment.

They are no longer able to care for themselves, and often require help doing the simplest tasks. Many end up in nursing homes.

About 10 percent of all Americans over age sixty-five have been diagnosed as suffering from Alzheimer's. Five percent of all cases occur in people as young as forty. Some forms of Alzheimer's are believed to be genetic; however, this disease can also strike people with no previous family history of Alzheimer's. As the baby boom population ages, the number of Alzheimer's cases will increase. As yet there is no cure and few effective treatments for Alzheimer's. Some drugs may forestall the progress of the disease, but they cannot stop it. We don't know how to prevent this disease, but there is one ray of hope, at least for women. Some studies have shown that menopausal women taking estrogen-replacement therapy can cut their risk of getting Alzheimer's by 40 percent.

One of the problems with finding a successful treatment for Alzheimer's is that the cause is still unknown. What researchers do know is that Alzheimer's is marked by an accumulation in the brain of a protein called beta amyloid. Many researchers believe that beta amyloid is responsible for the destruction of brain cells, which leads to Alzheimer's disease. A growing minority of researchers, however, now suspect that the formation of beta amyloid is actually a secondary symptom, and that the primary cause of Alzheimer's is a defect in the flow of blood through the small blood vessels in the brain.

Through the years there have been other culprits cited as the cause of Alzheimer's. For example, high concentrations of aluminum have also been found in the brains of Alzheimer's victims, and as a result some researchers believe that aluminum in the environment, such as aluminum cookware and aluminum compounds in deodorants could be a factor in this disease.

However, there is no scientific evidence that this is true.

What is the role of melatonin in the treatment of Alzheimer's? Several studies have shown that Alzheimer's patients suffer a disruption in their melatonin circadian cycle, and that this disturbance is often manifested in wakefulness at night. Alzheimer's patients often have a great deal of difficulty sleeping, and as a result so do their caregivers. Due to the lack of sleep, Alzheimer's patients often wander around at night, which is particularly dangerous because accidents are more likely to occur in the dark, or when someone is tired. Not surprisingly, their caregivers often suffer from both depression and sleep deprivation because they must be on call twenty-four hours a day. Caring for an Alzheimer's patient can be both physically and emotionally exhausting.

We feel that melatonin can be a boon to both Alzheimer's patients and their caregivers. In fact, we are about to undertake a study on the effect of melatonin on the sleeping habits and other deficits of Alzheimer's patients. The results won't be ready for some months, but we think that there is good reason to believe that melatonin therapy will help many Alzheimer's patients recover their normal sleep patterns. Melatonin is far superior to synthetic sleeping pills because it produces a better quality of sleep, and does not result in the morning hangover that sometimes accompanies sleeping pills. Melatonin may give those who are caring for Alzheimer's patients the security of knowing that their loved ones are sleeping soundly, in bed, and not wandering around, putting themselves at risk.

Although this has not yet been studied, we also theorize that melatonin may be able to improve memory in Alzheimer's patients. Sleep deprivation can lead to memory loss even in young, healthy people who do not have Alzheimer's. Therefore, we reason, it is possible that the restoration of sleep may help Alzheimer's patients retain better memory function.

Studies have also shown that Alzheimer's patients (like people with AIDS) have prolonged elevated levels of corticosteroids, the stress hormones discussed above. Corticosteroids can damage the hippocampus, the center of the brain responsible for the maintenance of memory. Melatonin has been shown to lower corticosteroid production. We therefore believe that it may also protect the hippocampus from corticosteroid-mediated stress damage and thus preserve memory.

Mental confusion can also be a sign of an underactive thyroid, which is also common among Alzheimer's patients and people who are generally depressed. As we explained in Chapter 3, melatonin helps regulate thyroid function. In young animals, thyroid hormone levels drop at night, indicating a slowing down of their metabolism, which is appropriate at times of rest. However, in older animals, thyroid hormone levels remain high at night. When we gave older mice melatonin, their thyroid hormone levels fell at night, just as they do in younger animals. In the mice that did not receive melatonin, thyroid function remained high at night, as would be expected in mice of their age. Clearly, melatonin has been shown to improve thyroid function, and we think that a side benefit of this may be improved memory and reduced confusion in Alzheimer's sufferers.

Many Alzheimer's patients may also be lacking a key vitamin involved in the production of tryptophan, the amino acid that is a precursor to melatonin. Starting at age fifty-five, about two thirds of all Americans have low blood serum levels of vitamin B_6, which is instrumental in the metabolism of tryptophan. Studies have also found that patients with Alzheimer's type dementia have low concentrations of substances leading to the production of tryptophan in their spinal fluid. Without enough of these vital substances, they are unable to produce enough tryptophan, which is later converted to serotonin, the precursor of melatonin. Quite possibly, many Alzheimer's patients may be suffering from a vitamin B_6 deficiency, which is also affecting their production of melatonin. Melatonin supplementation may correct this problem. Some people, however, may require an additional B_6 supplement.

Finally, in any discussion on Alzheimer's disease, it is important to note that some patients who are diagnosed with Alzheimer's may not have the disease at all. They may simply be profoundly depressed. Depression in the elderly can produce many of the symptoms associated with Alzheimer's, including memory loss, withdrawal from the world, and nighttime wakefulness. As of this writing, there is no definitive test for Alzheimer's, and distinguishing this disease from other mood disorders remains problematic. Therefore, it is important to note that many depressed patients show marked improvement when they are given antidepressants (such as monoamine oxidase inhibitors). For these patients, melatonin supplements may also help to restore their circadian melatonin cycles, and may relieve the insomnia.

ASTHMA

The more we learn about melatonin, the more excited we become about its many potential uses. For example, a friend of ours who has had asthma for many years swears that melatonin has helped to improve his condition. Asthma is a common respiratory disorder in which the air tubes of the lungs become constricted, impairing breathing. Asthmatics like our friend tend to have attacks that are often triggered by stimuli such as the presence of an allergen, an irritating chemical like pollen, exercise, or even stress. Steroid aerosol sprays that open up blocked airways are a common treatment for asthma, though not without chronic side effects in prolonged use.

At our suggestion, our friend has been taking melatonin regularly at night to treat insomnia. He says that melatonin not only has improved his sleeping habits, but that since he has been taking it he has noticed that when he works out at the gym his endurance on the treadmill has improved, and he has not felt the need to use his inhaler as often. We found our friend's observations to be so intriguing that we decided to see if any scientific research had been done on melatonin as an asthma treatment.

When we checked, we discovered an interesting study that had been performed in 1965, at the Hebrew University Hadassah Medical School and Cardiopulmonary Laboratory in Israel. In this study, the researchers tested the action of melatonin on the lungs of dogs. They found that when administered intravenously melatonin was an excellent bronchodilator, and appeared to work as well as some compounds that are commonly used for this purpose today. Although to our knowledge no one has pursued melatonin as an asthma medication, we think it looks promising and deserves more study. This is just one more example of how melatonin's use as a potential therapeutic treatment has yet to be explored.

DIABETES

Diabetes is actually a group of biochemical disorders characterized by the body's inability to utilize carbohydrates, sugars, and starches that are found in food. If carbohydrates are not adequately processed by the body, elevated levels of blood sugar may result.

Over time, this can lead to heart disease, kidney disease, stroke, and even blindness.

There are basically two kinds of diabetes. Type 1 or insulin-dependent diabetes—also called juvenile diabetes—occurs when the pancreas cannot produce insulin, the hormone that is instrumental in the breakdown of sugars and starches. Without adequate insulin, blood sugar levels can rise to dangerously high levels. People with insulin-dependent diabetes require daily injections of insulin. Insulin-dependent diabetes usually occurs before age forty, and accounts for about 10 percent of all cases of diabetes.

By far the most common type of diabetes, and the one that is a virtual epidemic in the United States, is called noninsulin-dependent diabetes. With this condition, sufferers become insulin-resistant. This means that although they produce enough insulin, their bodies do not utilize it efficiently. As a result, blood sugar levels can rise, and they can develop the same serious complications as result from juvenile diabetes. Insulin resistance is a prime example of how as the body ages it gradually loses its ability to adapt readily to its environment. Although the pancreas is still pumping out insulin, the insulin response has become sluggish and the patient is not responding to the stimulus of rising blood sugar. The older we are, the more likely it is that we will develop a form of insulin resistance. In the United States, about 15 percent of all people over age sixty-five have noninsulin-dependent diabetes. Obesity and a family history of diabetes are important risk factors; thus, maintaining normal weight is one of the best ways to reduce your risk of developing diabetes.

For those who have developed noninsulin-dependent diabetes, doctors typically recommend weight loss, diet, and exercise. Specifically, they recommend a diet low in refined sugar and high in certain types of easy-to-digest complex carbohydrates, such as are found in whole grains, legumes (beans), and vegetables. If you suffer from diabetes, you should be under the supervision of a physician and a nutritionist who can help you devise a diet plan.

Recently, insulin resistance has become a trendy disease. You may have read about insulin resistance in magazines and newspapers, or heard the term bandied about on popular talk shows. Some well-known diet gurus contend that insulin resistance is far more widespread among the general population than is generally believed, and that it is not primarily a problem of the elderly, but an affliction suffered by many people of all ages. These diet experts claim that the inability to break down carbohydrates can paradoxically lead to carbohydrate craving. In other words, the theory goes, since we are not utilizing carbohydrates properly, our bodies become starved for them and we consume more. Therefore, they conclude, obesity is actually a result of insulin resistance, because we are overeating to satisfy this carbohydrate need. To avoid this problem, they recommend severely limiting our intake of carbohydrates, including even the kind that are normally allowed for diabetics. This to us is an overly simplistic explanation of why so many people are overweight.

Although we have our doubts about the insulin resistance theory of obesity, we do appreciate the very real dangers of insulin resistance. We believe that melatonin may actually help prevent insulin resistance from occurring in the first place, and thus may help to prevent the occurrence of noninsulin-dependent diabetes. Insulin resistance is a concern in and of itself because high levels of insulin are known to accelerate hardening of the arteries. We also think that melatonin may provide other benefits to people who already have developed the disease.

We base our recommendations on studies that have

shown that people with diabetes produce less melatonin. We think that there may be a connection here; that the onset of diabetes may be influenced by the lower melatonin levels that occur as the pineal begins to wear out. Consider this: We know that melatonin helps to keep our hormones in balance, and that when melatonin production declines, our hormone levels may be disrupted. For example, during sleep, in addition to melatonin, we produce many other hormones, including growth hormone. Growth hormone can raise blood sugar levels, thereby promoting insulin resistance and diabetes. Melatonin helps to regulate the production of growth hormone. By normalizing growth hormone levels, it may help keep blood sugar levels in check and prevent diabetes.

Melatonin may also help to prevent diabetes in another important way, by regulating the production of corticosteroids. As discussed above, these stress hormones are released when we are upset, angry, or frightened. Corticosteroids increase the production of glucose, which in turn, raises blood sugar levels. This rise in blood sugar levels helps to rev the body up for action, and is part of our primitive flight or fight response. If we have to run across a savannah to escape a predator, all this blood sugar is put to good use. If, however, we are sitting at our desks or in our living rooms, producing corticosteroids because we are mad at a boss, or coworker, or relative, the blood sugar is superfluous and unhealthy. It just sits in our bloodstream until it is broken down by insulin. Interestingly, studies have found that diabetics have higher than normal levels of corticosteroids, which makes it more difficult for them to control their blood sugar. By controlling corticosteroid production and its subsequent rise in blood sugar, melatonin may help us avoid developing the internal hormonal environment that may trigger diabetes.

Down Syndrome

Although we do not usually recommend the use of melatonin for children, there is one exception to our rule. We believe that melatonin may be beneficial to children with Down syndrome in several important ways.

Down syndrome is the most common form of inherited mental retardation and is caused by a chromosomal abnormality. The risk of having a Down syndrome child increases exponentially with the age of the mother. Down syndrome can cause many physical problems that result in a shortened lifespan. Our interest in Down syndrome is twofold. First, one of us (Walter) has a nephew with Down syndrome, and, while watching him grow, he has been able to see firsthand the physical and emotional difficulties with which he and his parents have had to deal. Second, from a purely clinical viewpoint, we think that many of the symptoms of Down syndrome strongly resemble those of aging. For example, children with Down syndrome often have a weakened immune system, and as a result are especially vulnerable to infection. By middle age, they appear to be years older than their chronological age, and they are prone to develop some of the diseases associated with aging, such as osteoporosis and premature senile dementia. Similar to many older people, Down children also suffer from sleep disturbances. This is not only hard on the Down child, but it can be extremely draining for the parents, who are sleep-deprived because of the need to tend to a wakeful child. Caring for a child with Down syndrome requires a great deal of love and patience, and a good night's sleep can make all the difference between feeling completely overwhelmed and being able to cope with the demands of the situation.

We believe that melatonin may enable children with Down syndrome to sleep better, which in turn would reduce some of the stress experienced by their parents. In particular, melatonin helps to restore normal REM (rapid eye movement) sleeping patterns, which these children so desperately need. It is during REM sleep that we dream, and if we are regularly deprived of this sleep cycle we never feel rested, and irritability and even more serious emotional disturbances may result. Second, melatonin may provide a boost to Down children's weakened immune systems, which can help make them less prone to infection. As we have said, melatonin specifically stimulates the thyroid gland and the thymus gland, both of which are involved in the production of T cells, which is crucial for maintaining a strong immune system.

Children with Down syndrome have a subtle but significant deficiency in the mineral zinc. Like melatonin, zinc is crucial for the normal function of the immune system, and a zinc deficiency can lead to a corresponding deficiency in disease-fighting T cells. For some time, our friend and colleague Dr. Nicola Fabris of the Italian National Research Centers on Aging has been suggesting that zinc supplements could be of great benefit to Down children, by giving a boost to their suppressed immune systems. In fact, according to his studies, zinc can stimulate T cell production and correct many of the immune problems typically found in Down children. Zinc deficiency, however, is not always caused by an inadequate intake of this mineral. In addition, it may be caused by the inability of the body to utilize the zinc it has. In this case, supplements may not always be useful. Thus it is important to repeat that melatonin supplements, themselves, have been shown to normalize zinc levels.

We suspect that melatonin is involved in how zinc is absorbed and utilized in the body. Consequently, taking melatonin may help Down syndrome children to better utilize this essential mineral, and thereby strengthen their immune function.

PARKINSON'S DISEASE

In Chapter 1, we mentioned Emmy, Walter's former mother-in-law, a vibrant, energetic eighty-five-year-old woman who has been taking melatonin for over ten years. What we have found particularly interesting about Emmy's case is that when she began her melatonin treatments in 1984 she had already been diagnosed with Parkinson's disease. Parkinson's disease is known for its characteristic tremors or muscle spasms, which can be mild or severe enough to hamper mobility. It is very common among older people; indeed most of the elderly do develop some form of this disease. Some Parkinson's patients also suffer from an Alzheimer's-like syndrome in which they become forgetful and confused. When Emmy began taking melatonin (5 mg daily), her hands had already begun to shake uncontrollably, making it difficult for her to perform simple tasks such as writing or sewing. Today, Emmy is Parkinson's-free.

How could melatonin have produced this result? To understand the answer, you need to know a little about Parkinson's itself. Some cases of Parkinson's are caused by side effects from certain medications such as Thorazine, a tranquilizer, or some antihypertensive medications. When the medication is discontinued, the symptoms usually disappear. True Parkinson's, however, is caused by the malfunctioning of a particular group of brain cells called the substantia nigra that release a neurotransmitter called dopamine. In many patients, Parkinson's can be controlled by dopamine medications and other drugs, but these treatments do not stop the progression of the disease. Since melatonin has been shown to inhibit dopamine production, we might expect that it would aggravate Parkinson's symptoms. But studies have shown that in some, though not all, cases, Parkinson's patients improve when they take melatonin.

There is no proven explanation for this apparent paradox, but we theorize that melatonin has an action that is independent of dopamine. It's possible that melatonin somehow repairs or rejuvenates the cells in the substantia nigra, which could explain Walter's mother-in-law's amazing recovery. We have also postulated that melatonin may work indirectly, by stimulating the production of prolactin by the pituitary gland. Animal studies have shown that if prolactin is administered to rats that have a Parkinson's type disease, their symptoms quickly disappear. Since, depending on the circumstances, melatonin can boost or depress levels of prolactin, it may very well be that for some Parkinson's patients, melatonin can induce an increase in this hormone or improve the responsiveness to this hormone to produce a positive effect.

Melatonin's ameliorative effect on some cases of Parkinson's may be related, at least indirectly, to melatonin's antioxidant capacity. Parkinson's may be caused by a decline in the function of mitochondria, the tiny powerhouse within our cells that controls the production of ATP, the fuel that keeps the body running. As we age, we lose mitochondria, and quite literally run out of fuel. Mitochondria are particularly vulnerable to damage by free-radical scavengers, which, as we discussed earlier in this chapter, can destroy healthy cells. As a free-radical scavenger, melatonin may protect the mitochondria that inhabit the site of the brain that controls Parkinson's, and therefore prevent this disease.

VISION

Can melatonin help you maintain your youthful vision? There is substantial evidence that it can. As we have explained, melatonin is produced in three parts of the body: the pineal gland, the digestive tract, and the retina of the eye. The retina is a membrane at the rear of the eyeball that contains light-sensitive rods and cones that receive images formed by the lens of the eye. The retina in turn transmits the images through the optic nerve to the brain. We really don't know why melatonin is produced by the retina, or what function, if any, it performs in the eye. Our studies, and the studies of others, lead us to conclude, however, that melatonin may prevent many of the vision problems associated with age.

When we administered melatonin to old mice, we found that it had a rejuvenating effect on many organs of the body, and the eyes were no exception. Similar to humans, older mice typically develop cataracts, a cloudy or opaque covering that grows over the lens of the eye, which can cause partial or total blindness. If the cataract is severe, it must be surgically removed. Cataracts are one of the main causes of blindness among older people in the United States. The mice who had been treated with melatonin, however, did not develop cataracts. In fact, their eyes seemed to grow young with the rest of their bodies, leading us to conclude that melatonin had a restorative effect on their vision.

If you think about the many roles melatonin can play in the body, the fact that it may help prevent cataracts is not at all surprising. As we have discussed earlier, melatonin is, among other things, a potent antioxidant that can protect cells against damage by free radicals. Several studies have confirmed that antioxidants appear to protect against cataracts. For example, one major study conducted by the National Eye Institute and the Chinese Academy of Medicine in Beijing showed that antioxidant vitamins could reduce the incidence of cataracts in adults (ages forty-five to seventy-four) by 43 percent. Other studies have shown that people who eat diets rich in fruits and vegetables, which are abundant in antioxidant vitamins, also have a significantly lower risk of developing cataracts. There are also some animal studies that strongly suggest that melatonin has a protective effect on the eyes. Earlier in this chapter, in the section on AIDS, we referred to glutathione, an antioxidant found in many cells, including those in the eye. In one study, researchers gave newborn rats a compound that would inhibit the action of glutathione, and thus leave the rats vulnerable to damage by free radicals, which could cause cataract formation. One group of rats on the glutathione inhibitor was also given melatonin, and one group was given a placebo. After sixteen days, cataracts were observed in 100 percent of the rats treated with the glutathione inhibitor, but only 6.2 percent of the melatonin-treated rats developed cataracts. In fact, the rats on melatonin had much higher levels of glutathione than the untreated ones had. This indicated that the melatonin protected the glutathione from the action of the glutathione inhibitor, which in turn protected the rats from cataracts.

Glaucoma, another common eye disease, is the leading cause of loss of vision in the United States. Glaucoma is caused by increased fluid pressure within the eyeball, which can damage the optic nerve. In a study performed at the Departments of Ophthalmology and Psychiatry at Oregon Health Sciences University in Portland, researchers tested the effect of melatonin supplements on the fluid pressure within the eyes of humans. Although more research needs to be done, this study showed that melatonin reduced the pressure in the eyes, leading the researchers to conclude: "This may prove to be a therapeutically useful agent since melatonin appears to be relatively free of side effects and is effective in small quantities."

We have firsthand knowledge of one case in which melatonin completely reversed a serious eye disorder that primarily afflicts older people, and often leads to partial or even total blindness. Macular degeneration is a progressive disease that slowly destroys the macula, a part of the retina that is responsible for central vision. This is the kind of vision that is required for activities such as reading fine print, writing, or driving a car. Blind spots appear in the field of vision, and as the disease advances the blind spot can grow, although some peripheral vision usually remains.

Macular degeneration can occur on its own, or it can develop after surgery for a detached retina, another common eye problem of aging in which the retina becomes separated from its attachment. The retina is held in place by the pressure exerted by the fluid of the eye, but as we age the pressure can drop and the retina can easily become displaced and float around the eye. If this happens, the retina must be reattached by laser surgery. Even after the surgery, there is a risk that the retina will detach again. In fact, one of our friends in Milan had to have this surgery several times, and unfortunately, even though the surgery was successful, he then began to develop macular degeneration.

In this case, the loss of vision was a particularly

devastating blow to our friend, who as a teacher and a scholar was always either reading or writing, two activities that would be sharply curtailed by macular degeneration. In preparation for the dark days ahead, he had already begun to put his favorite books and papers on tape. At our suggestion, several years ago our friend began taking melatonin. After a few weeks, he reported that he had begun to notice a gradual change for the better in his vision. Within a few months, he said that his vision had returned. Wondering whether he was experiencing some kind of placebo effect, we declined to take his word for it. His ophthalmologist and later other doctors verified our friend's claim, confirming that he had indeed been cured and that this was the first time they had ever seen macular degeneration heal itself. Although the doctors did not quite believe that melatonin was the reason, they conceded they could offer no other rational explanation. Neither can we. Based on this event, clinical trials are now planned to determine whether melatonin could be an effective treatment for macular degeneration.

We do not know precisely why melatonin worked so well for our friend, but we suspect that it may have exerted more than one action in his eye. Melatonin may affect fluid formation, and thus normalize fluid pressure within the eyes, which in turn would protect against diseases such as macular degeneration. We also theorize that melatonin's capacity as an antioxidant may protect the macula from further damage. Melatonin may also affect the light-sensitive cells of the eyes in ways that we still do not understand. In the case of macular degeneration, melatonin's positive effect could also be related to the melatonin/zinc connection. As we have said, studies show that older people are often zinc-deficient and that melatonin normalizes zinc levels in both animals and humans. Zinc, in turn, may play an important role in the prevention of macular degeneration or retinal separation. One study performed at Louisiana State University Medical Center tested the effect of zinc on macular degeneration. In this study, patients with macular degeneration were either given zinc supplements or a placebo. The patients taking the supplements showed significantly less vision loss than those taking the placebo.

Although we don't have the definite proof yet, these studies and our own experiences have fully convinced us that melatonin can help preserve vision, and this deserves active controlled study.

Undoubtedly, as more attention is paid to the melatonin miracle, we will find even more uses for this remarkably versatile hormone. In this chapter we have discussed several diseases for which melatonin is likely to prove a useful therapy, but we believe that science has only begun to understand melatonin's true disease-fighting potential. Melatonin's potential to treat and heal is vast, yet that potential may go unrealized unless melatonin receives the attention from the research community that it deserves.

PART THREE

Nature's Sex-Enhancing Hormone and Other Benefits of Melatonin

CHAPTER 10

Melatonin and Sex

To us the discovery of the aging clock is most exciting not because we can extend life (which is exciting in and of itself), but because we sincerely believe this will make it possible for us to also enrich the quality of our lives so that we may fully embrace and fully enjoy life. Not just in youth, but for all of our years. What is tragic is to lose the physical strength and vigor that enables us to share in life's pleasures. It is not enough to extend life unless we can also extend our ability and our desire to enjoy it and to relish the very things that make us happy to be alive.

MELATONIN, HEALTH, AND SEXUAL VIGOR

We are all far too familiar with friends and relatives who, as they aged, grew increasingly sick and frail, and in the process grew ever more withdrawn from the mainstream of life. Too often, they lose interest in life, and, not surprisingly, in life-affirming activities, including the most life-affirming activity of all: sex. We think that one of the reasons for this is that people who are trapped in the downward spiral that has become the hallmark of aging are typically—indeed, logically—preoccupied with illness and disability. They lose a sense of their bodies as an instrument of pleasure, and as a result lose their interest in sex. It seems to us that one of the saddest things that can happen as we age is that we lose interest in sex, and that is why we are eager to point out that it need not be this way. By reversing this downward spiral, and by restoring strength and vigor, our work with melatonin suggests that it can help us prevent the decline in sexual energy that we now too readily accept as a natural consequence of aging.

You will recall from Chapter 3 that when we added melatonin to the evening drinking water of old mice (i.e., mice that were the equivalent of about seventy years old in human terms) it had a profoundly rejuvenating effect on them. Their coats grew thick and lustrous, their eyes remained clear and cataract-free, their digestion improved, and their strength and muscle tone was enhanced. They exhibited none of the wasting signs of aging that mice their age would normally show, nor did they develop the diseases that typically afflict mice of their breed and age. They lived to the human equivalent of one-hundred-plus years, and they appeared literally to grow young before our eyes. Their bodies showed none of the typical outward signs of aging, and they also maintained the strength and vigor of younger mice. They had both the appearance of much younger mice, and also exhibited the behavior of young mice as well. Both the males and females displayed, for example, the sexual fortitude of much younger mice, and they appeared to preserve interest in sex throughout their entire extended lifetimes.

Moreover, melatonin promises not only to maintain and to restore an interest in sex, but, our research has shown, it actually helps to rejuvenate sex organs. As our laboratory experiments confirm, melatonin prevents the atrophy of sexual organs that typically occurs as we age. In female mice, for example, as they age the ovaries shrink and eventually shrivel up. In male mice, there is also a shrinkage of the testes. The ovaries and testes are responsible for producing sex hormones, which, among other things, are involved in sexual drive. In mice taking melatonin, however, the female ovaries did not shrink as they normally do. In fact, mice as old as twenty-four months (the human equivalent of seventy to seventy-five) had the same size ovaries as much younger mice. Melatonin had the same beneficial effect on male sex organs. In male mice taking melatonin, the testes did not show any signs of shrinkage. We believe that there is a direct connection between the youthful state of the sex organs and the level of sexual activity, and all of these improvements were the result of melatonin supplementation.

HORMONES AND SEX

If you have ever had an erotic dream, you can thank your pineal gland. When your pineal gland is pulsing out melatonin, it induces the form of sleep known as REM (rapid eye movement) sleep, during which time vivid and intense dreams, including those of sexual content, occur. Similarly, if you have ever been sexually aroused, you should be grateful to your pineal gland. Sexual arousal occurs because your brain and your endocrine glands are pumping out sex hormones, and the activity of these glands is controlled by the pineal gland and its chemical messenger, melatonin. The same messenger is also involved in signaling cues that tell us to touch and cuddle, and hence is instrumental in the process we call bonding.

Libido, or sexual drive, is a complicated mechanism

that is as much connected to our mental well-being as to our physical state. The better we feel about ourselves generally, and about our bodies in particular, the more likely we are to be interested in sex. Clearly, by maintaining your body in a youthful state, melatonin can help maintain interest in sex. But libido is also regulated by hormones. In men, the male hormones testosterone and dehydroepiandrosterone among others, govern arousal and erection. In women, female hormones (estrogen and progesterone) and also male hormones, or androgens, are involved in the sex drive. In order to feel sexy, aroused, and interested, we need to produce normal levels of these hormones, and it is the duty of melatonin to make sure we do. Fluctuations in our melatonin levels stimulate the pituitary gland to release a number of hormones that regulate sexual activity. These hormones include luteinizing hormone (LH), which is involved in ovulation and the secretion of estrogen; follicle-stimulating hormone (FSH), which regulates the production of sperm in men and stimulates the maturation of the ovaries in women; and prolactin and oxytocin, which stimulate milk production and maternal bonding. The normal ebb and flow of hormones is essential to our ability to respond sexually. We believe that taking melatonin supplements at bedtime later in life, starting at the time when natural levels begin to drop, may help restore these other hormones to more youthful levels and thus enable us to maintain our youthful level of sexuality as well.

Melatonin can also make sex a more pleasurable experience at any age. Melatonin heightens the effect of endorphins, the natural tranquilizers produced by our bodies and that can, among other things, relieve pain and stress. The release of endorphins produces a sensation of pleasure and well-being. Endorphins are one of the reasons you enjoy a relaxed, soothing sensation after engaging in good sex. Melatonin's endorphin-enhancing ability, which increases the pleasure of lovemaking, becomes ever more important with each passing decade. As we age, we often lose our ability to experience pleasure. Physical ailments too often may distract us from savoring the special sensations of lovemaking. The older we are, the more vulnerable we are to the baleful effects of stress, and that too can interfere with the enjoyment of sex. Continual stress can make it impossible to relax and "go with the flow," which is a necessary part of enjoying sexuality or other pleasures of life. Through its effect on endorphins, melatonin can help relieve stress, and thus create an environment that is more conducive to lovemaking.

In addition to getting you in the mood for sex, melatonin may actually help to encourage the physical contact and intimacy that leads to sexual activity. We know that melatonin controls the production of two hormones in new mothers that trigger milk production, prolactin and oxytocin. As we have seen, these hormones also trigger a cuddling instinct in new mothers that impels them to cuddle and hug their newborn, promoting bonding between mother and child. Prolactin and oxytocin come into play not just in terms of mother-child bonding, but also play an important albeit subtle role in our sexuality. We believe that these hormones can provoke the same cuddling response in adults, and, at least indirectly, encourage sexual contact. In fact, studies have shown that when mice are injected with the hormones that melatonin regulates, these hormones produce a dramatic increase in the kind of behavior that we humans would describe as cuddling and hugging. Upon reflection, it strikes us as eminently reasonable that the same hormone that helps to establish the intense bond between mother and child would also contribute to the bond between its parents.

We are not surprised that melatonin would have such a dramatic impact on human behavior in light of the fact that melatonin regulates both ends of the human sexual cycle. A drop in melatonin levels ushers in puberty for both sexes, which marks the beginning of reproductive capability. A further drop in melatonin in midlife triggers menopause in women, the end of their reproductive capability, and the climacteric in men, the beginning of a decline in their sexual response.

Since melatonin helps our bodies retain their youthful state, many women have asked us if taking melatonin in midlife, before the onset of menopause, can extend fertility and delay menopause. With more and more women choosing to pursue careers in their twenties and thirties, the possibility of delaying motherhood until their forties or fifties or even beyond is an enticing one. We have not yet performed the studies necessary to determine with certainty whether melatonin can prolong fertility, but we have reason to believe that it may. We know that a drop in melatonin levels occurs at around the time menopause begins. We also know that melatonin has a rejuvenating effect on the body. Therefore we believe that one day melatonin may be used to extend the time that a woman can conceive and carry a child. However, since this is an area that is of such concern to women, it seems to us that there should be some well-run clinical trials to determine if melatonin can postpone menopause, how much melatonin is required to do this, and other pertinent questions.

MAINTAINING THYROID HEALTH

As we stated earlier, our ability to enjoy sex is often undermined by poor physical health. A common condition that can interfere with our enjoyment of sex involves the thyroid gland. The thyroid gland produces thyroid hormone, which regulates cell metabolism and reproductive function. About ten million American women—many of them young—suffer from an underactive thyroid gland, or hypothyroidism. This condition is three times more common in women than men, and is especially prevalent among people who are middle-aged or older. An underactive thyroid does not produce sufficient thyroid hormone, and this can result in depression, fatigue, susceptibility to infection, loss of libido, and infertility. Menstruating women who have underactive thyroid glands may experience heavier and more frequent periods. This is due to the failure of their ovaries to produce an egg every month, which results in a buildup of uterine lining. (When an egg is not produced, it is called an anovulatory cycle.) Hypothyroidism can be caused by problems of inborn metabolism, autoimmunity, iodine deficiency, or aging.

Thyroid deficiencies are also common among older people. This is one primary reason why older people have difficulty regulating their body temperature, and often feel too cold or too warm. We think that the loss of thyroid function and the consequent loss of energy could also be one of the reasons why older people lose their sex drive. When you don't produce sufficient thyroid hormone, your body doesn't have enough energy to produce or respond to adequate levels of sex hormones. Without the right levels of sex hormones, you can lose your interest in sex.

The typical treatment for an underactive thyroid is

to prescribe synthetic thyroid hormone, which usually cures the problem. In fact, many women who were infertile because of an underactive thyroid are often able to conceive after taking a thyroid supplement.

Melatonin helps to maintain the health of the thyroid, especially in older people, and may prevent hypothyroidism from occurring in the first place. Here's why. As we have explained in earlier chapters, the thyroid produces two hormones, T_4 and T_3; T_3 is a more potent form of the hormone, and thus provides more energy to the body. As the regulator of other hormones, melatonin is instrumental in the breakdown of thyroid hormone from T_4 to T_3. By keeping the thyroid gland active and functioning normally, it appears melatonin helps prevent the decline in thyroid function that occurs later in life and that can dampen sexual function and energy response.

MALE SEXUAL HEALTH

Melatonin may also help men retain their sexual potency by preventing a common medical problem that can interfere with sexual function, benign prostate hypertrophy or enlarged prostate. The prostate is a small, walnut-sized gland located between the bladder and the penis, above the rectum. The prostate produces semen, the fluid that carries sperm. More than half of all men over fifty develop an enlarged prostate in which, as its name suggests, the prostate gland becomes swollen. When the prostate becomes enlarged, it can interfere with both urination and sexual function. Although there are drugs that may relieve the problem, at least one in ten men will require surgical treatment, which can also result in sexual dysfunction. Melatonin may help to preserve the health of the prostate, and thus prevent this common ailment. Proscar, one of the drugs used to treat an enlarged prostate, works by inhibiting an enzyme (5-alpha-reductase) that breaks down male hormone into a more potent form that can stimulate the growth of prostate cells. Melatonin also inhibits this enzyme and thus may prevent the growth of prostate cells. In fact, in mice, when the pineal gland is removed, resulting in a decline in melatonin production, the prostate becomes enlarged. When melatonin is given as a supplement, however, the prostate returns to normal size. This is yet more evidence that melatonin has a positive effect on the health of the prostate.

Throughout this book, we have referred to the melatonin/zinc connection, and by that we mean that melatonin is instrumental in the transport and absorption of zinc in the body. Several studies have shown that melatonin supplements or pineal transplantation from a young mouse to an old mouse can restore low zinc blood plasma levels to their normal amounts. There are heavy concentrations of zinc in the male prostate. In fact a mild zinc deficiency can lead to a low sperm count. As we age, zinc levels tend to decline, and even if people do eat enough zinc-rich foods, their bodies may not be absorbing it properly. As a result, a proper zinc level becomes difficult to maintain. Melatonin appears to help restore and maintain normal zinc levels, and thus protect the health of the prostate.

Finally, melatonin may protect against a common condition that is one of the leading causes of impotency, and that is atherosclerosis, or the clogging of the arteries with plaque, a fatlike substance. In the chapter on heart disease, we discussed how melatonin helps to normalize blood cholesterol levels. High blood cholesterol levels are associated with the formation of fatty plaques in the arteries, the hoses through which blood travels from the heart to other parts of the body back to the heart. Every organ in the body requires an adequate blood supply to function normally, and the penis is no exception. If the blood flow to the penis is blocked due to atherosclerosis, it can impair a man's ability to maintain an erection. By helping to keep blood cholesterol levels normal, melatonin keeps the blood flowing everywhere that it is needed, including to the sex organs and brain, both of which must be operating in sync for sexuality to manifest itself.

KEEPING COUPLES IN SYNC

For couples, compatibility is the product of a number of factors, not the least of which is staying attuned to each other's daily cycles. Establishing the same rhythms as those of your partner, that is sleeping, eating, and waking at around the same time, helps to keep you in constant communication with each other. For many couples, this isn't an issue, but for some a lack of synchronicity can break up what would otherwise be a good relationship.

Not all of us can live according to the same schedule, but generally variations in schedules are not that extreme. Sometimes, though, differences in daily cycles are so extreme that they can drive partners to distraction. Some people are night people and feel wide awake and energetic into the wee hours. Others are day people and are ready to rise and shine just when the night people are hitting the sack. Obviously, when a day person and a night person unite, this can wreak havoc on a sexual relationship.

In situations where couples are being driven apart by differences in their daily rhythms, melatonin can be useful in helping them establish a pattern that puts them more in synchrony with each other. The night owl could readjust his bedtime by taking melatonin to induce sleep at an earlier hour. The day person could try staying up an hour or two later (which many people claim can actually make it harder to fall asleep) and use melatonin to induce sleep at the correct time. By using melatonin to reestablish sleep patterns, the couple could create a more harmonious relationship.

MELATONIN AS A CONTRACEPTIVE

Researchers have known for about a decade that melatonin regulates other hormones, including those that are instrumental in the menstrual cycle. In fact, the high levels of melatonin found in children are believed to suppress their sexual development. When these levels drop, puberty begins, and in girls ovulation commences. The possibility that melatonin can be used as an oral contraceptive had been studied by endocrinologist Michael Cohen, formerly of Dijkzigt University Hospital in Rotterdam. He has discovered that high doses of melatonin (75 mg daily) when combined with the female hormone progesterone can block ovulation. Today, the standard female contraceptive pill contains estrogen, a hormone that falls and rises monthly with the menstrual cycle. Estrogen has been shown to increase the risk of certain forms of cancer, including breast cancer, and though studies have been mixed, there is some evidence that estrogen birth control pills may increase the risk of breast cancer for long-term users. Because of the possible estrogen-cancer link, Dr. Cohen set out to develop an estrogen-free pill that would pose no cancer risk. Dr. Cohen, a cancer specialist, did research that gave rise to the melatonin/progesterone oral contraceptive, which contains 75 mg of melatonin and a small amount of synthetic progesterone, a hormone that is also involved in the menstrual cycle.

In Holland, more than two thousand women have taken the melatonin birth control pill for over three years, and the results have been very positive. The melatonin pill has proven to be every bit as reliable as the standard birth control pill but without any side effects. In fact, Dr. Cohen reports that the in-depth follow-up studies of more than three hundred women on the melatonin contraceptive show that women find the melatonin pill preferable to the estrogen pill for several reasons. First, unlike the estrogen contraceptive pill, which can cause headaches, bloating, and other unpleasant side effects, women on the melatonin pill report no side effects at all. Second, unlike the estrogen pill, which many women say tends to flatten out their cycles, the melatonin pill keeps their bodies more in sync with their natural monthly cycles. In other words, they feel the same monthly fluctuations in terms of mood and energy that they would feel if they weren't taking any contraceptive at all. Although this may sound strange, many women find it reassuring that a contraceptive is not interfering with their natural cycles. These women also say that unlike estrogen, which can suppress libido, the melatonin pill has enhanced their sex drive and improved their sex lives. (In light of what we just discussed, this comes as no surprise to us.) Finally, the women on the melatonin contraceptive pill also reported a generally heightened sense of well-being. In other words, melatonin made them feel better generally.

Through his company, Applied Medical Research, Dr. Cohen is currently seeking FDA approval to market this contraceptive in the United States. Clinical trials have been cleared to begin in this country shortly, and if things continue to go as well as anticipated, the melatonin contraceptive could be available here within a few years.

The high dosage of 75 mg daily is required only for

use as a contraceptive. It is important to note that for all other purposes described in this book, only a very small dose of melatonin is required, from as little as .5 mg daily for age reversal up to 5 mg to cure jet lag. (For specific information on dosages, turn to Chapter 14.) Still, it is significant and reassuring to see that even when melatonin is taken in very high doses, as is necessary to stop ovulation, it remains completely safe and without any negative side effects. Indeed, one of the surprises to us from Dr. Cohen's research is the finding that at such elevated dosages no sleepiness occurs in the subjects. Since at much lower levels melatonin is a powerful sleep inducer, we would have expected these women to complain of extreme drowsiness. As a result of Dr. Cohen's clinical trials in Holland, we conclude that at high dosages melatonin's effects as a sleeping agent is overridden. We speculate that melatonin works differently in very high doses than it does in lower doses, as do many other hormones.

MELATONIN AS A MENOPAUSE AID

Dr. Cohen's group is also testing a new type of hormone replacement therapy (HRT) for postmenopausal women that substitutes 75 mg of melatonin for the progesterone that is normally used in combination with low doses of estrogen. When a woman reaches menopause, there is a sharp drop in the production of estrogen, which can result in unpleasant symptoms such as hot flashes and insomnia. Due to lower estrogen levels, there is also an increased risk of developing heart disease and osteoporosis. Millions of menopausal women take hormone replacement therapy (HRT) to replace the lost estrogen. HRT has also been shown to diminish the unpleasant side effects of menopause and to protect against heart disease and osteo-porosis. Similar to birth control pills, HRT is most often prescribed in the form of a combination estro-gen/progesterone pill that is taken daily. Estrogen given alone can stimulate the buildup of blood in the uterine lining, which may increase the risk of devel-oping uterine cancer. However, progesterone encour-ages the lining to shed, similar to a monthly menstrual cycle, and thus protects against uterine cancer. The problem with progesterone, however, is that there are some indications that it may increase the risk of breast cancer in postmenopausal women. Therefore if mela-tonin can be used instead of progesterone, it could eliminate the risk of breast cancer and make HRT safer.

Melatonin's sex-enhancing effects are felt through-out our lives in many different ways. It is the hormone that ushers in puberty and "turns on" our sexuality. It contributes to the "cuddling" hormone that encour-ages hugging and bonding, which helps us to forge closer ties and more enduring relationships. By virtue of its age-reversing properties it can also help to pre-vent the physical problems associated with aging that often interfere with a satisfying sexual relationship. In short, melatonin is the sex-enhancing hormone that helps to promote a lifelong healthy interest in sex.

CHAPTER 11

The Stress-Relieving Hormone

A cover story in *Newsweek* magazine recently described the plight of Harvard University President Neil Rudenstine, who took a three-month sabbatical from his job because he was too exhausted to go on with his breakneck schedule. At the time that he decided to take a leave, Rudenstine was heading an ambitious million-dollar-a-day fund-raising campaign, a daunting task even by Ivy League standards. Rudenstine was under unremitting pressure. He was meeting with donors day and night, traveling from one alumni gathering to another, and also performing his other administrative functions. Reluctant to delegate responsibility, Rudenstine also micromanaged the university, getting involved in the smallest of details. After months of working at this intensity, Rudenstine realized that he was simply too burned out to continue to function at the frantic pace he had set for himself. Fearing that he was going to get sick, he knew that the time had come to take a much needed extended vacation.

The reason Rudenstine's crash caught our attention was not the fact that a brilliant and overburdened chief executive had succumbed to exhaustion. The story had resonance for us because we know he is not alone: Men and women from all walks of life, from salespeople to Post Office workers to homemakers, are succumbing to the unrelenting pressure of job and family responsibilities, and they are burning out. Few, however, are in a position to enjoy the respite of taking an extended sabbatical.

All these people are, to use an old but apt phrase, stressed out. Stress can be dangerous to our health. It not only inflicts emotional suffering, but can lead to physical damage, even death. According to the American Academy of Family Physicians, more than two thirds of all visits to the doctor are due to stress-related ailments, which include asthma, anxiety, headache, indigestion, fatigue, and nausea. Worker's compensation claims for stress-related ailments have increased 700 percent over the past decade. Numerous studies have documented the link between severe stress and gastrointestinal problems like colitis, heart disease, and even cancer. There is even growing evidence that diseases such as multiple sclerosis and rheumatoid arthritis may be triggered by a particularly traumatic or stressful event.

Moreover, there is nothing that ages us faster than chronic physical or emotional stress. Several years ago, *Longevity* magazine ran a photograph of a woman taken around the turn of the century. Her hair was gray. Her skin was sagging and wrinkled. Her eyes were sunken and looked worn. She looked like a withered, old woman. Astonishingly, at the time the photo was taken, this woman was only forty years old! The stresses of her life—which no doubt included multiple pregnancies, strenuous labor, coping with family illnesses such as whooping cough and tuberculosis—had taken their toll. It is no wonder that the life expectancy of women of her generation was but forty-seven years.

Today, at least in developed countries, improved

sanitation, immunization, and antibiotics spare us from many of the life-threatening illnesses that plagued our ancestors. Modern conveniences also spare us from much of the backbreaking labor that our grandparents knew. Our life span has increased accordingly. Yet life in today's world has its own stresses: workdays that begin early and end late; cellular phones and fax machines that allow us to take the office with us wherever we go; difficult bosses and demanding clients; alarm clocks and beepers that track our every move; air travel that allows us to attend meetings in three cities in one day; family and professional responsibilities to juggle; mortgages and tuition bills to pay.

No matter how far we might advance technologically, and perhaps because we are so technologically advanced, stress will always be a fact of life. It will also be a factor in how well and how long we live. Fortunately, melatonin can help protect us against the ravages of stress, and in this chapter we will show you how.

To understand how melatonin operates as a stress-buster, you first need to know a little about stress and how our bodies respond to it.

WHAT STRESS IS, WHAT STRESS DOES

The use of the word "stress" to refer to the anxiety-provoking things that happen to us and how we are affected by them was originated with a research scientist who borrowed the term from structural engineers.

Dr. Hans Selye, who began his career as a researcher at McGill University in Montreal in the 1930s, was an endocrinologist, someone who studies the endocrine system and the hormones that it produces. At the time, scientists knew very little about

197

the role hormones play in the body. Each gland was a new uncharted territory waiting to be explored. Selye was trying to learn about a particular substance that had just been isolated from the ovaries of animals. No one knew what this substance did, so Selye decided that he would give a group of rats daily injections of this ovarian extract to see if it had any effect. For his control group, Selye also injected other rats with a pure saline solution that contained none of the ovarian extract.

Several months later, Selye discovered that the rats that had received the ovarian extract had marked physical abnormalities. They had developed peptic ulcers. Their adrenal glands had become enlarged. Their immune system had been damaged. At first, Selye figured that all of this damage had been caused by the ovarian extract. Then, however, he examined the rats in the control group, which had not received the extract. He was astounded to find that they, too, had experienced the same type of damage.

Selye was completely thrown by these results. If the ovarian extract wasn't causing the physical changes, then what was? After giving the matter some thought, Selye theorized that even though the contents of the injections varied, both groups of mice had one experience in common: They all received daily injections. Selye reflected on the process of administering these injections, and realized that the rats did not enjoy them; in fact, they disliked them so much that often he had to hold them down to administer the shots as they squirmed and struggled to escape. Selye hypothesized that perhaps it was the sheer unpleasantness of continuous injections that had somehow triggered the physical changes in the body. Selye then devised all kinds of ways to make life unpleasant for rats. He kept them in cold rooms, he forced them to swim for their lives in cold water, he tied them up so that their movement was restricted, he subjected them to persistent loud noise. The rats that were subjected to these conditions all sustained the same bodily damage that the rats that had been injected in the earlier experiments sustained. To describe the unpleasant forces that inflicted the damage, Selye borrowed a term that had been used by structural engineers to describe the forces—load, high winds, earthquake—that assault bridges, buildings, and other structures. That term, of course, is "stress."

Humans, as we know all too well, are often subjected to stress. When we are, our body reacts in a number of ways. This stress response is regulated by our autonomic or involuntary nervous system, the same system that regulates such vital functions as the beating of our heart. The autonomic nervous system is divided into two parts, the sympathetic nervous system and the parasympathetic nervous system. The sympathetic nervous system regulates what scientists call our flight-or-fight response. This is a prehistoric response mechanism, and an example from prehistory is commonly used to describe it. When we are subjected to a stressful situation (for example, out picking berries and suddenly confronted by a hungry bear), a signal is sent from the brain's cortex to the sympathetic nervous system telling it to prepare the body for immediate action (for example, to run!). Our adrenal glands, located on top of our kidneys, start pumping what scientists call stress hormones, epinephrine and norepinephrine. These hormones in turn trigger a chain of reactions in which our body quite literally prepares for battle. Our blood pressure rises, our heart pumps faster, and the flow of blood is diverted from the digestive system and routed to the muscles where it is needed to fuel our escape. Our rate of metabolism rises as we consume more oxygen to fuel this activity. The pupils of our eyes dilate to let in more light to improve night vision. And, while all this is happening, yet another part of our adrenal glands begin producing other stress hormones called corticosteroids. Corticosteroids send blood sugar levels soaring to provide fuel to burn.

In sum, the flight-or-fight response gears us up for action. It gives us the burst of energy we need to run for our lives, or to stand our ground and fend off a predator. The mechanism was certainly useful back in the days of the cavemen, when pouncing lions, stampeding herds of mastodons, and warlike neighbors were facts of daily life. All this bodily revving up served a useful purpose—it saved our lives—and the stress hormones were consumed in the process.

Today, however, for most of us stress is a different experience. Few of us ever experience hand-to-hand combat, or stalk (or get stalked by) wild animals. Our days are filled not with wild animal predators but with ferocious bosses, difficult clients, surly cashiers, nasty divorces, and a maddening economy. To our brains however, it is all stress, and as soon as our brains perceive stress, they switch into battle mode and trigger the flight-or-fight response. The problem is that, for most of us, punching the boss or running away are not usually appropriate responses. Since we don't get to either fight or flee, the stress hormones stay in our bodies, where, over time, they can cause severe damage.

Stress hormones can injure every organ system in our body, from our hearts to our brains. Melatonin can blunt the negative effects of stress hormones, and by doing so can prevent a myriad of common diseases. In fact, many ailments that you may not even have thought of as being related to stress can in fact be caused by or exacerbated by stress. In this chapter, we will review how melatonin can protect us against the ravages of stress.

STRESS AND THE HEART

The heart is particularly vulnerable to the effects of chronic stress. Researcher Hans Selye, who as we noted earlier was the first to use the word "stress" in the medical context, found that continual exposure to stress could destroy portions of the heart muscle in mice, even mice who had no previous signs of heart disease. We're still not sure why this happens, but the effects of stress on the heart are very real. It is well documented that stress can kill heart cells, and if too many heart cells die, so can we. This aspect of heart disease, documented by Selye, gets little play today among cardiologists focused on atherosclerosis, but it is an area of clinical concern that deserves renewed attention.

Corticosteroids, one of the hormones produced in response to stress, appear to injure both the heart muscle and the arteries, the hoses through which blood flows to the heart and from the heart to the rest of the body. If our arteries become so impaired that they can no longer deliver an adequate blood supply, a heart attack may result. If the blood supply to the brain is impaired, it can cause a stroke.

Stress can also increase blood pressure, which can also inflict damage to the heart. Although the precise mechanism by which stress can raise blood pressure is not fully understood, we do know that when we are under stress the body begins to conserve salt and water to increase blood volume in the event of injury. If blood volume is reduced due to blood loss, your body won't be able to deliver enough oxygen and nutrients to the vital organs. The increase in blood volume requires an increase in blood pressure to help the heart pump the extra fluid.

Melatonin has been shown to blunt the negative effects of corticosteroids. It does this by normalizing levels of corticosteroids in our body, preventing them from becoming too high. Thus melatonin can protect our hearts and blood vessels against the damage inflicted by stress.

STRESS AND DIABETES

Prolonged exposure to corticosteroids can raise blood sugar levels so that we have the fuel to fight or flee. However, continual peaks in blood sugar levels can also increase the risk of developing diabetes. Indeed, medical science has long known that people with diabetes have higher than normal levels of corticosteroids. Diabetes is not only a serious disease in its own right, but it can increase the risk of developing heart disease, stroke, and blindness. Once again, melatonin may help to prevent stress-induced diabetes by curbing the effect of corticosteroids, thus preventing the continual rise in blood sugar levels.

STRESS AND OSTEOPOROSIS

We do not think of osteoporosis as being a stress-related disease, but continual exposure to corticosteroid stress hormones can weaken the bones and leave them vulnerable to breaks and fractures. Osteoporosis, a condition common in older women, is characterized by thin, brittle bones. Complications from injuries that occur as a result of osteoporosis—for example, broken hips—are one of the leading causes of death among older women. How does stress affect the health of bones? Corticosteroids have been shown to block the growth of special cells on the end of bones that are necessary for the formation of new bone cells. By controlling the levels of corticosteroids, melatonin may help prevent this insidious disease associated with hip fractures, premature disability, and even death.

STRESS AND BRAIN FUNCTION

Stress hormones can also damage the brain and can even affect our capacity to think clearly and remember information. In fact, corticosteroids have been shown to injure cells in the hippocampus, the portion of the brain that controls short-term memory. As we age, we typically lose some of our ability to retain new information. For example, it becomes harder to remember names and faces of people with whom we have been recently introduced, and it may take longer to process and absorb new facts. Perhaps this loss of short-term memory is due to a lifetime exposure to stress. Some researchers even suspect that Alzheimer's disease, which results in a loss of short-term memory, may be due to damage of the hippocampus, and that, in turn, may be linked to severe stress and the prolonged exposure to corticosteroids. Here again, melatonin's positive effect on decreasing corticosteroid response can help to protect our brains from stress-induced damage.

STRESS AND THE IMMUNE SYSTEM

Long-term exposure to corticosteroids that are produced during stress can also suppress the immune system. Many studies have documented that stress can reduce the number of white blood cells, which are necessary to fight against disease. For example, several research studies involving soldiers in combat-like situations have shown that their immune systems were significantly weakened, leaving them vulnerable to infection. One of the reasons why this happens is that extreme stress can block the production of thyroid hormone, which is essential for every major body activity, including the production of disease-fighting immune cells. There is also evidence that stress hormones can actually damage the immune cells themselves, thus preventing them from doing their job effectively.

In the laboratory, we re-created the effect of stress by giving animals an injection of corticosterone (the animal form of corticosteroids) and then checking for their immune response. We found that the corticosterone depressed the production of disease-fighting antibodies by 60 percent. In other words, these animals were ill-prepared to defend their bodies against disease, and the same is true for humans who are under stress.

Earlier, when we discussed immune function, we showed dramatic examples of how stress can erode immunity and leave us vulnerable to disease. For example, when an animal is exposed to severe stress, its thymus gland, the gland where the important disease-fighting T cells are stored, begins to shrivel and disappear. When these animals were given melatonin after being exposed to the stressful situation, their thymus glands were rejuvenated, and so was their immune function. We have other even more dramatic examples of how melatonin can counteract the damaging effects of stress. In another study, we injected a high dose of corticosterone (stress hormone) into mice and not surprisingly, the animal's immune response was severely depressed. In this weakened state, these animals would have fallen prey to the first infection that came their way. However, we then gave the same animals an evening injection of melatonin. Literally, overnight, their immune system quickly bounced back to normal. This is yet more evidence that melatonin can block some of the damage inflicted by stress hormones on the immune system.

Melatonin not only bolsters the immune system against the malign effects of stress by controlling corticosteroids, but actually works with special stress-relieving chemicals that are produced by the immune system. These chemicals are called endorphins, and they are natural painkillers that are produced by both the brain and immune cells. Endorphins not only help relieve pain, but can help reduce anxiety and promote a feeling of euphoria. Melatonin has been shown to enhance the effect of endorphins, and by doing so helps the body withstand the stress of illness.

THE EFFECTS OF STRESS WORSEN AS WE AGE

Stress is hard on people of all ages, but the older we are, the greater its toll. As we have seen, stress can inflict physical injury to people of all ages, but as we age, these injuries become more difficult to withstand.

As we mentioned earlier, when we are under stress, our bodies produce corticosteroids, which can cause severe damage to many of our body systems. Among other things, corticosteroids can injure heart muscle, raise blood sugar to abnormally high levels, destroy thyroid function, inhibit sexual response, and even dampen our immune response. In older people, corticosteroids remain higher for longer periods of time than they do in younger people. As a result, when we are older our bodies are flooded with these harmful stress hormones for longer periods, and are therefore more vulnerable to damage. What makes stress even more insidious to the elderly is the fact that organ systems are beginning to decline and can't tolerate any additional damage by corticosteroids. For example, the immune system is already weaker and less capable of waging battle against foreign invaders. The thyroid gland has also begun to wind down. The heart must now work harder to pump blood throughout the body. This decline in body systems leaves an older person even more susceptible to the negative effects of stress.

As we age, each stressful situation that we encounter triggers a physical response in our bodies, upsetting our physical and mental equilibrium. In other words, it throws us off balance. When we are young, we are able to bounce back. When we are older, we become more inflexible, or set in our ways, not just in terms of our mental outlook, but also in terms of our body's ability to respond to change. Each assault on our psyche takes a deeper and more lasting toll. We are both physically and emotionally less equipped to recover after an illness, a sad event, an argument, a disappointment, or even a relatively benign stress such as a change in lifestyle. This is not to say that some young people are not rigid and inflexible. In fact, some of them may act older than people who are chronologically old enough to be their grandparents. Yet certainly on a physical level, there is a difference in how we cope with stress in youth and in old age.

We believe that this general weakening of our bodies that leaves us vulnerable to stress is attributable to a loss of pineal function and a drop in melatonin levels. Thus there is an antidote to the devastating physical effects of stress on our aging bodies, and it is melatonin. It can neutralize the harmful effects of stress by restoring the natural hormonal balance that is eroded by constant exposure to stress. Melatonin can restore thyroid function, which provides us with strength and resilience to meet new challenges. It can restore thymic immune function and minimize the dangerous effects of corticosteroids, which can cause untold harm if left to their own devices. It can even help prevent the sleep deprivation that is caused by anxiety. (For information on how melatonin can cure insomnia and sleep disorders, see the following chapter.) By normalizing hormones that are out of control, melatonin can help to restore a sense of control and empower us to withstand the rigors of daily living.

CHAPTER 12

Nature's Own Sleep Aid

If you have trouble sleeping, you are not alone. About one third of all American adults, some fifty million people, suffer from sleep disorders at one time or another. "Sleep disorder" is an umbrella term that experts use to describe everything from insomnia to frequent night wakenings. Sleep disorders can be brought about by acute stress, alcohol abuse, or medical problems such as heart disease or ulcers. But sleep disorders can also strike for no apparent reason, especially after we reach middle age. We are especially vulnerable to disrupted sleeping patterns as we grow older—about one half of all Americans over the age of sixty-five experience some form of sleep disorder. Sleep disorders are also a common side effect of menopause. It is not unusual for a menopausal woman to be abruptly awakened by a hot flash, or to suffer from insomnia. The fact that older people and menopausal women are plagued by sleep problems is no coincidence. In both cases, melatonin levels have started their decline, and the disruption in melatonin cycling makes getting a good night's sleep difficult.

Melatonin (which, as you now well know, is produced by the pineal gland at night) plays a critical role in helping us to fall asleep and stay asleep through the night. Melatonin supplements can normalize sleep patterns, and sleeping well is absolutely critical to a restorative and rejuvenating rest. In this chapter, we will show how this safe, nonaddictive hormone can help you solve your sleep problems, and why melatonin is far superior to any other so-called sleeping pills.

THE IMPORTANCE OF SLEEP

Whether your problem is that you have difficulty falling asleep at night, or that you sleep fitfully, or that you wake up too early, your problem is serious and not to be taken lightly.

We say this because science has taught us that sleep is essential for our physical and emotional well-being. The failure to get sufficient sleep can adversely affect virtually every system of the body. Sleep deprivation can seriously undermine the functioning of the immune system, making us vulnerable to infection. It can prevent our brains from functioning normally, interfering with our ability to focus and think clearly. It can hamper our ability to manage stress and thus it can promote anxiety. It can make us depressed and impair our judgment. It can make us just plain irritable. In fact, there are few aspects of daily living that are not disrupted by sleep deprivation.

In order to understand why sleep is important, and how melatonin can help improve our sleep, we need to review what sleep actually is and why we do it.

Sleep has two purposes. The most obvious one is to allow our bodies to rest and refuel. Many of our body systems wind down while we are sleeping. Our heart rate drops and so does our blood pressure. Our metabolism, the process by which our body uses energy, switches into low gear and our body temperature drops. This is not to suggest that important things are not happening in our body while we are sleeping, and this point takes us to the second purpose of sleep. Although during sleep our mind and body are, in a sense, at rest, they are, in another sense, hard at work. Since during sleep we are far less demanding on our organ systems than we are when we are awake and active, sleep is the time when our body's cells can concentrate on repairing themselves and creating new cells. This repair work is essential for the maintenance of a strong, healthy body, and if we don't get enough sleep, your internal "body shop" is not able to do its extraordinarily important job.

So that you will fully understand the restorative nature of sleep, here is an example of what happens to just one system, your immune system, when you miss a single night's sleep. As we mentioned earlier in the chapter on immunity, in a test conducted by Dr. Michael Irwin, a psychiatrist at the San Diego Veterans Affairs Medical Center, twenty-three healthy men ages twenty-two to sixty-one spent four nights in a sleep laboratory. They were allowed to sleep normally for the first two nights, but on the third night they were denied sleep between 3 A.M. and 7 A.M., which is considered prime slumber time. Dr. Irwin found that the activity of "killer cells," the type of immune cell that fights off viral infections, fell significantly in eighteen of the men the morning after the sleep loss, indicating that as a result of sleep deprivation their body's ability to fend off infection was diminished. Fortunately, the level of immune cells returned to normal after the volunteers were allowed to sleep through the next night uninterrupted. Dr. Irwin demonstrated the devastating effect on just one system of the body caused by only one night of lost sleep. Now magnify this effect over all the other body systems and you can see that sleep loss can pose a serious threat to health, especially if it occurs over a prolonged period of time.

CIRCADIAN CYCLES

When we sleep, and to some extent how well we sleep, is governed by our circadian cycle, the day-night cycle that controls the activities of plants and animals, including humans. The circadian cycle is about twenty-four to twenty-five hours in length, similar to the twenty-four-hour day. In this cycle, our body is governed by dozens of interrelated cycles of internal clocks, all of which are working together to synchronize us both internally as well as with one another and the world around us. Internal rhythms control and coordinate our hormone production, hunger, moods, body temperature, and our energy level. An internal clock also controls our sleep/wake patterns.

The pineal gland and the hypothalamus, another gland in the brain, work together to control the sleep/wake cycles of our body. The pineal gland, triggered by the dark of night, releases melatonin. When this occurs our body temperature lowers, our heart rate decreases, and we surrender our bodies to a more restful state. The level of melatonin in the blood peaks between 1 and 5 A.M. Then, as morning's light approaches, the secretion of melatonin is inhibited. What is happening is that light is entering our brain through pathways that extend from the retina of the eye to a point in the hypothalamus called the superchiasmatic nucleus and onward to the pineal gland. When the pineal gland receives this light signal, it knows that it is time to slow down the production of melatonin. Thus the pineal gland's ability to detect light and dark is essential for maintaining our circadian rhythms. The fact that the light/dark signals are transmitted to the pineal through the retina of the eye may explain why some blind people experience a disturbance of sleep/wake cycles. That disturbance, and the attendant variation in the secretion of melatonin, is probably due, at least in part, to a lack of light/dark perception.

It has been well documented that when people are deprived of outside light and mechanical clocks, they eventually lose track of time, including all sense of whether it is day or night. They may fall into lengthier sleep/wake patterns that can last as long as thirty-three hours, but meanwhile their biological clocks, which should keep them warm in the middle of the day and cold at night, may keep cycling on a twenty-four- to twenty-five-hour schedule. As a result of these non-synchronized systems, there is an uncomfortable feeling of imbalance and disorientation.

Melatonin does not merely affect the rhythm of our sleep. It also profoundly influences the kind and quality of sleep we experience. As you will see, there are different types of sleep, and they follow a predictable pattern.

The brain is extraordinarily active during sleep. We can actually measure this activity by a special medical test called an EEG, which tracks changes in brain waves. If you looked at an EEG of brain waves during sleep you would see two distinctive patterns of brain wave activity. First, there is the nonrapid eye movement activity or NREM. Second, there is the rapid eye movement activity, or REM. Each type of activity is produced by a different type of sleep, and each type of sleep performs different functions.

NREM sleep is generally regarded as the most restful kind of sleep. During NREM sleep, breathing is slow and regular, blood pressure is low, and there is very little muscle movement. There are four stages of NREM sleep. When we first go to sleep we're in the transition stage between wakefulness and sleep. Then we progress downward, to stage 2, a light sleep. During stages 3 and 4, also known as delta sleep, our brain activity is recorded in large, smooth, slow waves.

These are generally believed to be the most deeply restful phases of the sleep cycle.

During the time of peak melatonin production, we are more apt to experience REM sleep, or "faster" sleep, which is recorded in shorter, faster waves. During REM sleep, we dream, and our body behaves as if it were awake, with peaks and troughs of psychological, physiological, and biochemical activity. Our heart and respiratory rates fluctuate, and although our eyelids are closed, our eyes move rapidly. Our eyes seem to be following a fast-moving object or scanning a book or crowded room. This indicates that we are dreaming.

SLEEP CYCLES

A pattern of NREM and REM sleep repeats itself in predictable sequences throughout the night, forming a constant series of sleep cycles. Each cycle consists of between sixty and one hundred minutes of NREM sleep followed by a shorter period of REM sleep. At the conclusion of the REM sleep period the cycle is complete. At this point there might be a brief period of arousal during which we might open our eyes briefly, turn, or shift position slightly.

We typically have four to six sleep cycles per night. NREM sleep accounts for about 80 percent of our total sleep. With each sleep cycle, however, the amount of time spent on REM sleep increases. During the first cycle, REM sleep may be as short as five minutes, but during the last cycle REM sleep may stretch to thirty to sixty minutes.

Certainly we need to get adequate sleep, the precise number of hours of which are particular to each person. But what is of especial importance to us all is the kind of sleep we get or miss out on. While stage 4 NREM is the most restful kind of sleep, evidence points to the fact that dreaming REM sleep is of paramount importance.

There are many theories as to why. Some people believe that REM sleep and dreams allow us to cope with and work out the day's threatening or upsetting experiences in a way that our conscious minds cannot. According to this theory, dreams provide an outlet for the impulses we seek to suppress during the day, allowing us to discharge these instinctual drives safely. Others think REM sleep dreams allow us to perform a sort of mandatory clean-up of data our brains need not address, while neatly filing away the important information. One scientific study indicates that REM sleep plays an important part in learning and consolidation of memory. After animals were given various learning tasks, they experienced increased periods of REM sleep. Similarly, researchers found that in humans REM sleep increased several days after the subjects had been exposed to intensely demanding and stressful events. Researchers also found that subjects who were deprived of REM sleep had trouble learning.

But whatever the reason REM sleep is important, it's clear that if we don't get enough of it we may experience serious negative physical and psychological changes. We may suffer increased appetite, loss of appetite, irritability, anxiety, and difficulty concentrating. REM sleep is so important that when we are deprived of it our brains try to compensate for the loss by producing more REM sleep. This process is called compensatory dreaming by sleep researchers. They report that after a period of deprivation, REM sleep may increase up to 40 percent, for several days, before winding back down to normal levels.

WHEN CIRCADIAN RHYTHMS
GO OUT OF WHACK . . .

Maintaining normal sleep/wake cycles is essential to our general well-being. When these cycles are disrupted, serious sleep problems can result. For example, in one sleep disorder called delay sleep phase syndrome, sufferers have a slow circadian rhythm, which makes it extremely difficult for them to experience sleepiness at the right time. Sometimes they do not fall asleep until three or four in the morning. In the case of another disorder, advanced sleep phase syndrome, the sufferers fall asleep as early as 8 P.M., and awaken in the wee hours. This is a problem that affects great numbers of elderly people. Yet another disorder, the nontwenty-four-hour sleep/wake cycle, causes sufferers to stay awake for tremendously long periods of time and sleep for prolonged periods, creating a cycle that can last up to fifty hours.

In all three cases, chronotherapy, a body-clock-resetting technique, provides a careful shift to a more socially acceptable schedule and a healthier, restorative sleep pattern. Chronotherapy involves using light to restore normal circadian rhythms. Researchers have found that short intervals of exposure to bright light can trick the internal clock into a more regular sleep pattern. They suggest, for instance, that night owls, or those people suffering from delayed sleep phase syndrome, benefit from a half hour walk in bright sunlight soon after waking. There are many theories as to why exposure to bright light can normalize circadian rhythms. Although there are no clear answers, it seems obvious that many of these sleep disorders are caused by an erratic flow of melatonin and that exposure to light must somehow normalize the production of melatonin.

As we explain below, taking a melatonin supplement is another effective way to reset the body clock to regain a normal circadian cycle.

MELATONIN AS A SLEEP AID

When melatonin was first isolated in the late 1950s by researchers Lerner and Case, it was found to have a mild sedative effect in animals. In 1982, Richard Wurtman, a pioneer in melatonin research, demonstrated that melatonin can induce sleep in humans. In his initial experiments at the Massachusetts Institute of Technology's Clinical Research Center, Dr. Wurtman used very high doses of melatonin (240 mg), and he found that these high doses made his subjects too tired to function normally the next day. However, more than a decade later, in a groundbreaking study, Dr. Wurtman found that even very low doses of melatonin were capable of inducing sleep. In his study, Wurtman administered between 0.1 and 10 mg of melatonin to twenty subjects before bedtime. All subjects reported an increase in sleepiness and all of them slept longer. Wurtman found that subjects who took melatonin fell asleep in five to eight minutes, while those receiving a placebo took an average of twenty-five minutes to fall asleep.

Tiny doses of melatonin are sufficient to bring melatonin blood levels to their normal nighttime levels and to induce sleep. Because melatonin does not produce the dependency or side effects that sedatives, tranquilizers, or sleeping pills do, it holds great promise as a substitute for them. In 1990, a National Institutes of Health panel issued a report that concluded that sleeping pills—both prescription and over-the-counter—

are overused and addictive. The panel urged the medical research community to concentrate on the underlying cause of insomnia rather than the symptoms. That is precisely what melatonin does. It corrects the imbalances in the body's circadian rhythm that prevent a good night's sleep. Moreover, people who have used melatonin as a sleep aid say that it produces a more refreshing sleep than that produced by sleeping pills.

There are many different types of medications used to treat insomnia. These include tranquilizers, antidepressants, and the class of drugs known as hypnotics, also known as sleeping pills. Most of these drugs have serious drawbacks. Some of them can raise blood pressure, some can cause hangoverlike effects, and some are addictive. All can interfere with normal sleep cycles, that is, and thereby disrupt the pattern of REM and NREM sleep. Other sleep-inducing drugs adversely affect the quality of sleep. Ironically, in the long term, conventional sleep-inducing drugs actually perpetuate sleeplessness by disrupting natural sleep rhythms.

RESTORING HEALTHY SLEEPING PATTERNS

Many people over age sixty have difficulty sleeping. While this segment of the population comprises only about 14 percent of the population, they consume up to 45 percent of all sleep medications.

A frequent syndrome among people of advanced years is to find themselves falling asleep shortly after dinner, and then waking very early in the morning. Many complain that this too-early-to-bed and too-early-to-rise schedule can isolate them from the mainstream of life. Although they may try to readjust their schedules, they are usually unable to do so on their own. These changes in sleep patterns experienced by the elderly are caused by a shift in circadian rhythms that is caused by a reduction in nighttime melatonin production. As a result, nighttime cycles go awry. When we are younger, our bodies are programmed to rouse us from sleep by a rise in body temperature that occurs around daybreak. However, in our later years, a shift in hormonal cycles produces a rise in body temperature as early as three or four o'clock in the morning. This revving up makes it extremely difficult to stay in a relaxed sleep state.

Melatonin plays an important part in restoring these people to an internal rhythm that is more in sync with the world around them.

A recent Israeli study reports that a slow-release form of melatonin can prevent insomnia in older patients. Conducted at the Technion Medical School in Haifa, the study found that men and women between the ages of sixty-eight and eighty who took melatonin had less trouble falling asleep and slept longer without waking up. The time required to fall asleep was cut by more than half, from forty minutes to fifteen. In addition, the subjects reported that they experienced a more refreshing sleep.

This is important news, because as we advance in years, we are increasingly susceptible to toxic drug reactions, including overreactions to sleep-inducing drugs. This results not just because of frequent use but because many older people also take other medications. The combination of sleeping pills and other drugs poses an increased hazard for the elderly, further complicated by changes in bodily function that go hand in hand with aging. As we age, we tend to absorb and excrete medication more slowly. Our nervous systems may also become more sensitive, and this could exacerbate the effect of combining drugs. In addition, narcotic sleeping pills may cause older people to stumble or fall if they get up at night, or feel groggy or hungover in the morning.

At best, conventional sleeping pills have only limited usefulness. They provide a temporary solution to insomnia. There is mounting evidence that melatonin may be a more effective, and certainly a safer, alternative to sleep problems, whether the problems involve the amount or quality of sleep a sufferer is experiencing. It is nonaddictive and, once it has had its synchronizing effect on the circadian cycle, its use can be discontinued but its benefits will remain. Melatonin is the only "sleeping pill" that actually can correct the physiologic problem that is causing the sleep disorder. Once the underlying problem is corrected and normal sleep cycles are restored, melatonin is no longer needed. It may in the future become necessary intermittently to reset your internal clock if and when it again goes awry.

TIPS ON HOW TO GET A GOOD NIGHT'S SLEEP

Whatever your sleep problem, melatonin will almost undoubtedly help you achieve a restful sleep. Since melatonin works by resetting your internal clock, it treats the underlying cause of your sleep problem, which is the disruption of the natural sleep/wake cycle. Therefore, melatonin should correct any number of sleep disorders, including insomnia, frequent night awakenings, and waking up too early.

For all sleep disorders, we recommend taking between 1 to 5 mg at bedtime to restore normal sleep patterns. The effect of melatonin will vary among individuals. Some people may find that the smaller dose will be sufficient for them to achieve a good night's sleep. Others will need a higher dose. To determine the exact dosage that is right for you, we recommend that you begin with 1 mg at bedtime. If you find that you sleep well with just 1 mg, continue to take that dose for subsequent nights. If your problem is not solved, for example, if you find that you are still waking up frequently at night, increase the dose the subsequent nights by 1 mg (up to 5 mg) until you determine the dosage that best enables you to sleep properly and feel refreshed in the morning.

If your problem is insomnia and you find you are not falling asleep with the initial 1 mg dosage, you may increase your dose by 1 mg. If you're still awake, you can continue to increase your dose by increments of 1 mg every twenty minutes until you reach a maximum 5 mg.

If you find that after taking melatonin at night you awaken feeling groggy in the morning, this is a sign that your bedtime dose is too high, and you need to reduce it.

Even once you are sleeping well, we recommend that you continue to take melatonin for two weeks to ensure that you have reset your body clock and reestablished your natural sleep pattern. After that time, most people find that their internal clock has been corrected, and they no longer need melatonin to sleep. (For more information on how to take melatonin, see Chapter 14.)

By taking melatonin at bedtime, you can practically guarantee a good night's sleep and also restore your normal sleep cycles. Yet in addition to taking melatonin when you have a problem, here are some other things you can do that will help you maintain a normal sleep cycle:

- Regular exercise will benefit sleep, but not right before bedtime. Physical exertion at night tends to stimulate instead of relax your systems.

- Establish a fixed sleep schedule, then stick to it. (Take your melatonin at approximately the same time each evening.)
- Use your bed for sleeping. Don't use it to watch TV, pay bills, or chat on the phone. Reserving the bed for sleep will help your body get in the mood for sleep when you go to bed.
- Get out of bed when you open your eyes in the morning. Don't hit the snooze button. Spending time falling in and out of sleep will interfere with the regulation of your biological clock and you'll end up feeling groggier.
- If you have more than occasional insomnia don't spend time in bed waiting to fall asleep. If you're spending nine hours in bed but sleeping only five of those hours, try going to bed an hour later every night and set the alarm a little earlier. By the end of the week the sleep you get will be more concentrated and refreshing.
- Don't smoke. Nicotine stimulates the nervous system and interferes with sleep. In some sleep laboratory studies, smokers experienced far greater difficulty than nonsmokers falling asleep, but found their sleep patterns improved when they abstained.
- Find a pillow you like! Backache, neckache, or excessive sneezing could indicate your pillow is not the right density or content for you.
- Keep the noise down. If you live on a busy street, consider double-glazing or insulating. Move your bed away from the window. Carpeting, heavy drapes, and sound-absorbing tiles can also add a measure of peace. Soothing sounds, such as the steady quiet drone of an air conditioner or cassette tapes of white noise like rain or surf can also help.

221

• Establish a ritual/cue. You may need not just physical but also psychological cues that it's time to sleep. Try to do the same relaxing, no-stress activities every night before bed. Read a boring book, water the plants, check for locked doors, or flip through a favorite travel book.

CHAPTER 1 3

Getting Back in Sync:
Tips on Overcoming Jet Lag
and SAD

Our circadian rhythm is the day/night cycle that regulates our major life-sustaining activities, including when we sleep, when we wake, and when we eat. Our body is governed by dozens of interrelated cycles produced by "internal clocks," which work together to synchronize us to the world around us. Internal rhythms control and coordinate our production of enzymes and hormones, which in turn control hunger, mood, body temperature, and energy level.

The pineal gland is key to maintaining the normal functioning of our internal clocks. It works in sync with another body clock, the suprachiasmatic nuclei, a cluster of nerve cells situated in another key center of the brain, the hypothalamus. Each day, light that passes through the eye sets the timing mechanism of the pineal gland. At night, the pineal gland interacts with the suprachiasmatic nucleus, sending messages alerting our body that it is dark. The pineal gland, aware of darkness, begins to secrete melatonin. The fluctuation in melatonin regulates the day/night cycles. Other hormones working in sync with melatonin con-

trol our body's other rhythms. Light suppresses melatonin production; therefore, the duration of daylight,
and even seasonal changes in day length, can affect
the ebb and flow of melatonin.

At times, our natural body cycles may be disrupted.
Traveling across time zones, for example, can cause
jet lag, a common complaint that is triggered by a disturbance in day/night cycles. Seasonal affective disorder (SAD) is another common problem involving a
disruption of circadian cycles that occurs in temperate
climates during the winter. People with SAD are sensitive to the lengthened periods of darkness in winter,
which can alter their melatonin cycling, and create
psychological and physical problems associated with
depression. In this chapter, we will discuss how and
why we fall out of sync, and what to do to get back on
track.

JET LAG

Jet lag is a recent phenomenon. At the turn of the
century, the mere suggestion that we could zoom
across time zones faster than our bodies could adjust
to the time change would have seemed like a scenario
straight out of Jules Verne. Now that jets have replaced trains and cruise ships as the most common
mode of long-distance travel, skipping time zones has
become commonplace. So has jet lag. And as any frequent flyer will tell you, jet lag can be hell.

It's interesting to note that migrating animals, many
of which trek tens of thousands of miles each year, are
careful to stay within their time zones. Perhaps they
intuitively know that crossing time zones can wreak
havoc on their bodies, and the same is true for humans. If you've ever stayed up all night cramming for
a final exam or completing a special project at work,

you know how confused and disoriented you feel after even one sleepless night. The next day, you may have difficulty remembering things, feel hungry at inappropriate times, have difficulty regulating your body temperature, be short-tempered, and in general, feel off balance. If you don't sleep when your body expects to sleep, wake when your body expects to wake, and eat when your body expects to eat, you can throw all of your body systems out of kilter. This is precisely what happens in the case of jet lag. When we travel cross-country or across oceans to another continent, it can take several days for our bodies to adjust to the new schedule. In fact, the rule of thumb is that it takes the body a full twenty-four hours to recover for every time zone that you cross. For example, if you cross the five time zones between New York and London, you will need on average five days to recover. Jet lag can be particularly hard on businesspeople who need to arrive at their destination fresh and able to think clearly, and on vacationers who don't want to spend several days of their holiday feeling out of sorts.

Since the 1980s, scientists have begun to take a serious look at the causes and possible treatments for jet lag. Our friend Josephine Arendt at the University of Surrey in Guildford, England, has pioneered many of these early studies. Dr. Arendt was one of the first researchers to explore the use of melatonin as a means to prevent the symptoms of jet lag. Familiar with melatonin's role in regulating sleep/wake cycles, Dr. Arendt reasoned that melatonin should be able to reset the body's biological clock to help it adapt more quickly to a new time zone. After hundreds of experiments on human subjects, Dr. Arendt's research strongly suggests that people who take melatonin suffer far fewer symptoms of jet lag than those who don't and bounce back faster after long trips. Similar studies by other researchers confirm Dr. Arendt's results.

The Melatonin Miracle

Word spread rapidly of melatonin's positive effect on jet lag among frequent fliers. Publications from *The Wall Street Journal* to *Vogue* magazine to *Business Week* have focused on this particular use for melatonin, and today countless numbers of people use melatonin to prevent jet lag. We both travel a great deal ourselves, and find that melatonin does the trick for us.

When you travel across time zones, take 3 to 5 mg of melatonin prior to bedtime once you are in your new destination. If you wake up in the middle of the night and are unable to fall back to sleep on your own, take another 3 to 5 mg to make yourself drowsy. Continue to take melatonin at night until you have fully reset your body clock (which usually takes about four days). When you return home, readjust your body clock by taking 3 to 5 mg of melatonin before your normal bedtime. Most people find that by following this simple regimen they no longer experience the symptoms normally associated with crossing time zones.

In addition to taking melatonin, here are some other simple things that you can do to avoid jet lag:

- Drink plenty of fluids while in the air to replace the fluids that are lost due to high altitude and changes in air pressure.
- Avoid alcoholic beverages, as they can further disturb your already disrupted sleep cycles by interfering with your melatonin cycling.
- Avoid coffee and caffeinated beverages such as colas, which can also interfere with sleep and contribute to dehydration.
- Try to get enough exercise in your new destination. Often, when we're traveling, we don't walk

or exercise as much as we do at home. The lack of activity can also contribute to sleepless nights.

• Take your meals at local time when you arrive at your destination. Digestion also helps the brain to accelerate its adaptation.

WINTER DEPRESSION

SAD is an acronym for seasonal affective disorder, a form of mood disorder that is triggered by the change of season or, perhaps more specifically, by the shortened days of fall and winter. Beginning from as early as September and lasting through March in the Northern Hemisphere, SAD victims are unable to adjust their body rhythms to the decreased exposure to daylight, becoming physiologically, and ultimately emotionally, distressed and out of sync. Many experts now believe that the depressive symptoms associated with SAD are due to a shift in the circadian rhythm caused by a form of biological malfunctioning that occurs in response to the shorter and darker days of fall and winter. Since it is the pineal gland that is responsive to light, and its secretion of melatonin a key factor in the regulation of the circadian and related cycles, SAD research is now concentrating on the critical interplay among light, melatonin, and other fluctuating rhythms that regulate body chemicals.

SAD strikes about 1 percent of the population, and is three times more likely to affect women than men. This comes as no surprise to us. Women's lives are more governed by biological cycles (such as the menstrual cycle) than are men's, and therefore are more likely to be vulnerable to the negative effects of a disruption in their biological rhythms.

Although as far back as Hippocrates' time physicians have observed a seasonal change in mood, SAD was not officially recognized as a mood disorder until the early 1980s. Dr. Norman E. Rosenthal, a researcher with the National Institutes of Health, was the first to identify SAD and establish a link between a particular pattern of behavior and the onset of winter. According to the *Diagnostic and Statistical Manual of Mental Disorders,* the official guide to psychiatric disorders, there are some specific criteria for a seasonal pattern disorder:

- There is a regular relationship between the onset of major depressive episodes and a particular time of the year.
- The individual experiences a full remission or release from depression at a characteristic time of the year.
- In the last two years, two major depressive episodes have occurred that demonstrate the relationship between the episode and the season, with no episodes having occurred outside of that time.
- Seasonal major depressive episodes outnumber the nonseasonal episodes over the individual's lifetime.

One of the most predominant features of SAD is a seasonal change in eating habits, usually seen as an increase in appetite that prompts a craving for carbohydrates. Typically, most of us do experience a change of diet during the colder months, eating more hot dishes, such as noodles or chili, and cutting back on salads and fruits because of the limited variety of available fresh produce.

This doesn't sound particularly extreme. But for SAD patients, the dietary changes are more specifically related to mood. They report an increased intake of pasta, bread, pastry, potatoes, chips, chocolate, and candy during the winter months. Their intake of caffeinated beverages also rises substantially.

When asked why they chose these foods, hunger was never the driving force, but rather the selection was consciously made to combat tension, anxiety, or mental fatigue. After eating, in fact, the majority of SAD sufferers reported feeling calm and clearheaded.

There is a physiological basis for this. Carbohydrate-rich food appears to accelerate the production of serotonin, a hormone produced by the pineal gland that carries signals across the gaps between brain cells. Serotonin is also a precursor to melatonin, which means that it is converted to melatonin as the body needs it. Serotonin is believed to play an important role in alleviating some forms of depression and is the key mediator affected by Prozac, our most popular and effective antidepressant.

Along with carbohydrate cravings, there are a number of other key symptoms of SAD. Between 1981 and 1985, the National Institute of Mental Health surveyed over fifteen hundred patients with SAD and developed a statistical profile of the disorder. Among the findings:

- Ninety-six percent of SAD patients reported decreased activity in winter.
- Ninety-four percent stated that interpersonal problems—relationships with spouses, lovers, family members, friends, and coworkers—occurred during these months.
- Ninety-six percent noted feelings of sadness, 84 percent experienced anxiety, and 79 percent reported increased irritability during the winter months.
- Difficulties at work were mentioned by 88 percent.
- An increase in appetite and an overall change in body weight was noted. More than seven out of ten patients experienced an increase in weight.
- More than six out of ten patients reported their sexual drive had dropped.

- Some patients found that their symptoms of depression improved dramatically as they traveled closer to the equator, where the amount of night and day is equal.

While some symptoms of SAD are found in other forms of depression, the particular combination of lethargy, anxiety, irritability, and dietary changes matched up against the seasonal changes present a specific disorder.

It is clear that SAD is caused by the disruption in the cycling of hormones and body chemicals that govern the circadian rhythm, to which the exposure to light is key. Exactly how or why this interruption occurs in some people and not in others is still under investigation.

As we mentioned earlier, most of our bodily functions, including physical activity, sleep and food consumption, water intake, and body temperature operate on the circadian rhythm cycle. So, too, do the levels and cycling of crucial hormones and enzymes, which can profoundly affect mood.

The control of these rhythms is in large measure a function of the timing and duration of our exposure to bright light. Researchers are now exploring the relationship between symptoms of depression as they are connected to fluctuations in body chemicals, and most particularly melatonin.

The Role of Melatonin

Although the cause of SAD is not known, research so far suggests that SAD is triggered by a seasonal disruption in the cycling of melatonin, which throws the circadian rhythms off balance. In the majority of patients with SAD, melatonin does not fluctuate normally throughout the night. Under normal conditions, melatonin should peak at around 2 A.M. and then begin to fall. Studies have found that in SAD patients, however, melatonin levels remain high for about two hours longer than normal, and then begin to drop.

It has been well documented that when melatonin levels are abnormal, either too high or too low, it can result in symptoms related to psychological disorders. For example, recent research has shown that melatonin levels are abnormally increased in people with manic disorder (subject to extreme mood swings), and yet are abnormally low in people with some kinds of depression. There is in fact a "low melatonin syndrome" in depression. The syndrome is characterized by low melatonin levels and disturbed circadian rhythms governing the production of stress hormones.

Evidence does seem to suggest, however, that erratic secretion of melatonin is only one mechanism that produces the main symptoms of SAD. At this point it isn't clear whether melatonin is directly involved in causing SAD or whether abnormalities in melatonin secretion are simply a by-product or a marker of the illness.

The Therapeutic Role of Light

Researchers have learned that the farther north the area (in the Northern Hemisphere), the higher the incidence of SAD. In fact, latitude, the distance from the equator, is found to be the most important geographical element in determining the severity of the disorder. One recent study found that 25 percent of the population in northerly latitudes is affected by at least some of the SAD symptoms. This is especially true of weight gain and excessive daytime fatigue. Also, farther north, where the darker days of winter begin earlier, SAD symptoms appear earlier and remit later in the year than they do in climates closer to the equator, where the seasonal light remains constant.

In the northeast section of the United States, symptoms usually appear in late October or November and begin to remit in February or March. In contrast, the farther south toward the equator you go, the depressive episodes begin later and remit earlier.

The issue of course with latitude has to do with the way sunlight strikes the earth. The farther north one travels the more diffuse the sunlight. The less sunlight, the higher the rate of SAD.

A survey conducted by the newspaper *USA Today* revealed, not surprisingly, that states with higher northern latitude, a greater number of cloudy days, and generally lower temperatures reported the highest incidence of SAD. Some studies show that Northerners are ten times more likely than others to develop a case of SAD.

Sharp changes in geography can even exercise significant influence over the triggering of SAD within very short periods of time. SAD patients report upon leaving a winter region and traveling to Florida that within days their mood lifts significantly. Upon returning to their home, they are plunged back into a depression within a matter of days.

For people who are hypersensitive to changes in light, travel can disrupt the critical balance of their circadian cycles.

The effect of light on mood has long been recognized by the medical profession. It wasn't until 1980, however, that light therapy became a recognized technique. Dr. Norman Rosenthal (the researcher who first identified SAD) was aware that melatonin produces seasonal changes in the behavior of many animals. He began to consider the possibility that melatonin might play a significant role both at the onset and in the severity of the disorder.

Dr. Rosenthal explored what would happen if patients with SAD were exposed to bright light during depressive episodes. He found that the impact of light, both in terms of the speed and completeness with which it relieves SAD symptoms, was dramatic.

A persuasive explanation for the profound decrease or elimination of SAD symptoms with exposure to light is that it helps to reset the biological clock that governs the secretion of melatonin. Research has also shown that for those SAD sufferers who have melatonin rhythms that are delayed as compared to normal patients, bright light advances the time of onset of melatonin secretion.

Other researchers had similar results. Peter S. Mueller, a psychiatrist at the National Institute of Mental Health, reviewed in the early 1980s the emotional and geographical history of a twenty-nine-year-old woman he had been treating for cyclic bouts of winter depression. He noted that the farther north she traveled, the earlier the onset of depression and the longer she stayed depressed into spring. That this was indeed a pattern was supported by the fact that when she journeyed to Jamaica during the winter months her depression disappeared within a couple of days of arrival. Mueller postulated that sunlight might be contributing in some way to the woman's depression and decided to experiment with light therapy.

Light, he knew, has two effects on melatonin rhythms. It can reestablish the melatonin rhythm (daytime, through the use of light, can artificially be reversed with night) and it can suppress melatonin secretion entirely (if dark periods are eliminated).

On consecutive mornings he exposed the patient to 2,500 lux of supplemental full-spectrum light (1 lux is equal to the light emitted by one candle). The patient recovered from her depression within a few days.

Through the use of light, Dr. Mueller had found a way to reset the woman's circadian cycle.

Michael Termon of Columbia University has found that exposing SAD patients to 2,500 lux for two hours in the morning brings complete remission from both depression and carbohydrate craving in roughly half of SAD sufferers, and usually after only a few days of treatment. Dr. Termon also thought it may be possible to enhance the efficacy of treatment by increasing the amount of time patients are exposed to light or by increasing its intensity. Dr. Termon's group has recently developed a new computerized device that SAD patients can use at home that simulates natural light.

Due to the large number of SAD sufferers, there are numerous centers springing up around the country that offer bright light therapy. For information on where to find a physician near you who specializes in the treatment of SAD, contact the psychiatric department of your local hospital or medical school.

SAD and jet lag are examples of what happens when our natural cycles are disturbed. When our bodies are working well, we are unaware of our circadian rhythms and the extent to which we are still under the influence of nature's biological clock. When our circadian cycles are disrupted, however, we feel the full force of nature's influence on our lives. We feel out of sync and out of touch with the rest of the world. It is then that we most intensely feel the profound role that these natural cycles play in our lives.

CHAPTER 14

How to Take Melatonin: The Right Dosages

In *The Melatonin Miracle,* we have shown the extraordinary range of benefits that melatonin can offer.

- **Age reversing:** Melatonin can extend our lives by decades while keeping our bodies "young."
- **Disease fighting:** Melatonin can help prevent heart disease, cancer, and other common diseases.
- **Stress relieving:** Melatonin can protect us from the destructive effects of chronic stress.
- **Cycle restoring:** Melatonin is a safe, nonaddictive sleeping agent that can cure disruptions in our sleep/wake cycle, such as jet lag and insomnia.

Melatonin works in tandem with the pineal gland, the body's regulator, to monitor and govern our other body systems. When the pineal gland falters, whether the failure is due to a disruption in circadian cycles from jet lag, or the breakdown in pineal function due to aging, melatonin will help to boost our regulator back to its peak capacity. If the pineal gland is working well, so does the rest of the body. When the pineal gland is out of whack, it throws our other body systems off balance.

So how much melatonin do you need to take in

order to get your body back in sync? The question of when you should take melatonin and how much to take will depend on the problem that you are seeking to correct. The regimen that we recommend for age-reversal is markedly different, for example, from our recommendations for curing jet lag or insomnia. In this chapter we will break down into separate sections the guidelines for dosage information and instructions for taking melatonin according to each of the specific problem areas that melatonin addresses.

But first, we want to set some general guidelines and commonsense precautions. We are basing our recommendations on studies of how melatonin naturally works within our bodies. While other scientists in the field may recommend much larger doses than we are suggesting, it is our belief that, to gain the optimal benefits of melatonin, more is not necessarily better. We are aiming to approximate the balance of hormone levels that naturally occurs when we are youthful and in our peak health. To artificially boost our melatonin level above that youthful level is not in keeping with our program.

Bearing in mind that while the principle that over-arches all of our thinking is to restore melatonin to our youthful level, we do not recommend melatonin supplementation for children. The reason is simple. In childhood melatonin production is already at its highest level and therefore it need not and should not, except in very special circumstances, be boosted higher.

We also do not recommend melatonin supplementation to women during pregnancy and lactation. The reason for this is again very simple. In pregnancy, the mother is already naturally transmitting melatonin to the fetus via the placenta, and to increase the mother's melatonin level would in turn increase the amount delivered to the fetus, which is something we do not recommend.

MELATONIN FOR AGE REVERSAL

Our melatonin replacement strategy is to restore your melatonin level to what it was when you were in your twenties. We use this value as our baseline, because, when we are in our twenties, our melatonin blood level is at its adult peak of about 125 picograms. After that, the level drops off very gradually, until we reach our midforties, when a dramatic decline in our melatonin production occurs. This decline steepens with each passing year, so that by the time you are eighty, your melatonin level is half what it was when you were in your twenties. Our strategy therefore is to reverse this downward curve and maintain our melatonin level at its constant, youthful peak. Doing this is not complicated. All that is necessary is to take the amount of melatonin required to bring your level up to its youthful baseline. That means you only need to take a small dose in your forties, a slightly larger dose in your fifties, more in your sixties, and so on. By restoring your melatonin to its youthful level we restore the function of your body's aging clock—the pineal gland—and help maintain your body in the youthful state. (A dosage chart is printed on the next page.)

We know from research that in most people, the level of melatonin begins its most precipitous adult decline at about age forty-five, so this is a good time to begin your melatonin replacement therapy. However, not all of us fit into this norm. Depending on our genes, this falloff may begin earlier or even later. If you have a family history of what we call the diseases of aging, such as cancer, cardiovascular disease, and heart disease, beginning melatonin replacement as early as your thirties or early forties may help you overcome a genetic predisposition to these problems.

Although it is unnecessary for younger adults to begin an age-reversing program with melatonin, and we do not recommend it below the ages we specify, it is fine for adults of any age to use melatonin to cure other problems. If you are an adult of any age, including a young adult, who wants to treat jet lag or a sleep disorder such as insomnia, for example, you may take melatonin on a short-term basis to resolve those specific problems. (See dosage instructions for jet lag and sleep disorders.)

We don't believe that by starting replacement therapy earlier than we recommend that you can get a head start on reversing the aging process. Nor should those of you who are in your fifties or older think that if you haven't already started taking melatonin by the time you were forty-five that you have missed the boat. On the contrary, by restoring melatonin levels to their youthful peaks you can produce age-reversing benefits no matter when you begin.

How Much Melatonin Do You Need?

To maintain your melatonin levels at their youthful peaks, we recommend the following dosages at the following ages. These dosages are based on normative levels of melatonin in adults as they age and the amount of supplement required to restore levels to their youthful peaks.

Age	Dose of Melatonin
40–44	Take .5 to 1 mg at bedtime
45–54	Take 1 to 2 mg at bedtime
55–64	Take 2 to 2.5 mg at bedtime
65–74	Take 2.5 to 5 mg at bedtime
75 plus	Take 3.5 to 5 mg at bedtime

You will notice that we consistently recommend that melatonin be taken at bedtime and that the dosage increases with age. For most people, melatonin induces drowsiness and it is best to take it just before sleeping. If you find that the recommended dosage leaves you groggy in the morning, that means the dosage is too high for you and we recommend that you reduce it by approximately .5 mg at a time until you find the right level for you.

When you go to your health-food store or pharmacy, you will find that melatonin comes in capsules and tablets, typically in strengths of 2, 2.5, and 3 mg. If the right dosage for you is lower, simply do the following:

For tablets: Break a tablet to the size that you need. For example, if you have a 2 mg tablet and you want a 1 mg dose, break the tablet in half. If you want to take a .5 mg dose, break the tablet into quarters.

For capsules: If you have a 3 mg capsule and want to take a 1 mg dose, empty the contents of the 3 mg capsule into a small dish. For the first dose, mix approximately one third of the contents with an ounce of liquid. (Store the remaining contents in a small, covered dish in the refrigerator.) For the second dose, mix approximately one half of the remaining melatonin with an ounce of liquid. For the third dose, mix the remaining melatonin with an ounce of liquid.

Walter takes his nightly 5 mg dose of melatonin with a teaspoon of wine or cognac, which, he believes, helps the body to absorb it more rapidly because melatonin is quickly solubilized with alcohol. (This does not mean that you should take melatonin with a full shot of liquor before bedtime. In fact, alcohol can interfere with your natural ability to cycle melatonin. However, a teaspoonful will not have any adverse effects.) If you prefer, you can also divide the contents of a 3 mg capsule into thirds and put each third into an empty gelatin capsule, which can be purchased at the drugstore.

Melatonin is also available in a sublingual form that dissolves under the tongue and is absorbed by the body more rapidly.

When to Take Melatonin

This is very important: Melatonin should only be taken at night, before bed. Remember, as darkness falls, it tells our pineal gland to release melatonin, which in turn tells our body that it's time to sleep. Therefore, it's not surprising that most people will find that melatonin makes them somewhat sleepy. Thus we recommend that you take melatonin about a half hour before bedtime. If you are a night-shift worker, your daytime bedtime, rather than the usual nighttime, governs when you take your dosage. After taking melatonin, don't engage in activities that require a state of alertness, such as driving or operating machinery. Although melatonin will not make you feel "drugged" in the way that a narcotic sleeping pill does, you may feel relaxed and drowsy and ready for sleep.

Does It Matter Which Brand to Buy?

There are a variety of companies producing melatonin, and it is readily available in most health-food stores and many pharmacies. Different brands offer different doses in their capsules or tablets. There are two forms of melatonin available: (1) the synthetic forms, and (2) the so-called natural melatonin, made from the extract of animal pineal glands. We prefer and recommend synthetic melatonin. Your pharmacist or shopkeeper will help you select the correct product.

Can I Take Melatonin If I'm Already Taking Hormonal Replacement Therapy?

Yes. Millions of postmenopausal women are taking hormonal replacement therapy (HRT) to replace the estrogen that is lost when the menstrual cycle stops. Although some women take estrogen alone, today most women take a combination of estrogen and progesterone. Some women take HRT for a short time simply to alleviate some of the more unpleasant symptoms of menopause, such as hot flashes and insomnia. However, many women are now taking HRT indefinitely because it has been found to help prevent heart disease and osteoporosis, two of the most common medical problems of older women.

Some women have expressed concern about taking both estrogen and melatonin. They are worried that melatonin will somehow block the action of HRT, or that the HRT will interfere with melatonin. We don't think there's anything to worry about. These hormones coexist in a young woman's body without causing any problems, and there's no reason why they shouldn't work as compatibly later in life.

MELATONIN FOR DISEASE PREVENTION

Although we generally do not recommend beginning your melatonin regimen before age forty-five to reap its age-reversing benefits, there may be special circumstances that make it advisable to start melatonin therapy as early as your thirties. Melatonin, as we have explained, is a disease-fighting hormone, and in that role may help prevent two of the most common diseases associated with premature aging and death: heart disease and cancer. If you are at high risk of developing heart disease—if you have a parent who has had a heart attack before the age of fifty, or you have problems such as high blood pressure, or high cholesterol, which increase your risk of having a heart attack—we believe it is advisable to start your melatonin supplementation at a younger age. Additionally, if you are at high risk of developing cancer, or have cancer, it may also be beneficial to start melatonin replacement therapy earlier, since cancer patients' values are lower than normal. In view of Dr. Russell Reiter's observations, preventing a drop in melatonin levels may help protect you against carcinogenic action.

We think that preventing a drop in melatonin levels will help you overcome these genetic predispositions. If you do have a family history that is worrisome, you might want to consider asking your physician to do a comprehensive blood test to measure certain "vital statistics" next time you go in for a physical examination. For example, your physician should check all blood lipids, including cholesterol and triglycerides. Your physician should also check glucose levels to see if you are utilizing insulin correctly, and liver enzymes to check for liver function. If your chemistries show evidence of abnormalities, then you might want to consider starting the age-reversing regimen with melatonin earlier.

Apart from the general usefulness of a blood workup as a diagnostic tool, it will also give you a baseline for measuring the benefits of melatonin supplementation. As we age, there are notable changes in the blood levels of many of these important lipids, enzymes, minerals, and vitamins. We believe that melatonin replacement therapy will restore many of these substances to their youthful levels.

MELATONIN FOR SLEEP

Melatonin is an excellent, natural sleeping aid. Since melatonin works by resetting your internal clock, it treats the underlying cause of sleep problems, which is the disruption of the natural sleep/wake cycle. Therefore, melatonin should correct any number of sleep problems, including insomnia, frequent night awakenings, and waking up too early.

For all sleep disorders, we recommend taking between 1 and 5 mg at bedtime to restore normal sleep patterns. The effect of melatonin will vary among individuals. Some people may find that the smaller dose will be sufficient to achieve a good night's sleep. Others will need a higher dose. To determine the exact dosage that is right for you, we recommend that you begin with 1 mg at bedtime.

For Insomnia

If the problem you are trying to resolve is insomnia, and you are unable to fall asleep within thirty minutes after taking your 1 mg dose of melatonin, then you can increase your dose from 1 to 2 mg the same night. If 2 mg doesn't work within ten to fifteen minutes, then increase your dose by another 1 mg (which will bring you up to 3 mg total). If you're still awake (which we seriously doubt), you can continue to increase your dose by increments of 1 mg every twenty minutes until you reach a maximum of 5 mg.

Once you have determined the dosage that works best for you, repeat that dosage on subsequent evenings at bedtime. Although you will now be enjoying a good night's sleep, we recommend that you continue taking melatonin at bedtime for two weeks. By continuing with melatonin for two weeks you are thereby resetting your body clock and reestablishing your natural sleep schedule. As a result, after two weeks, when you stop taking melatonin, even without melatonin at bedtime you will continue to sleep well.

For Restless or Disturbed Sleep

If your problem is that you wake frequently during the night or that you wake up very early and cannot fall back to sleep, melatonin can also help. Again, you should start with 1 mg of melatonin at bedtime. If your sleeping problem was not resolved that first night, if for example, you found that you still woke frequently in the night, or if you woke too early and could not fall back to sleep, then increase the dose on the next night by 1 mg (making a total of 2 mg). If your sleeping problem is still not resolved, you can continue to increase the dose on subsequent nights by 1 mg (up to 5 mg) until you are sleeping properly and feeling refreshed in the morning.

Once you have found the dosage that works best for you and you are sleeping restfully through the night, we recommend that you continue taking the melatonin for two weeks. This allows you to reset you body clock and to reestablish your natural sleep pattern. That will help to ensure that even after you stop taking

the melatonin at the end of two weeks, the sleep benefits will remain.

Note: If you find that after taking melatonin at night
you wake up feeling groggy the next morning, that is a
sign that your bedtime dose is too high, and you need
to reduce it. (For more information on melatonin and
sleep disorders, see Chapter 12.)

If you are already taking melatonin daily as a
part of our age-reversal therapy, is it all right to
take additional melatonin for insomnia or other
problems sleeping? Yes. Just follow the same instructions listed above. (Do not exceed a total of
5 mg daily.)

Melatonin for Jet Lag

Jet lag is caused by a disruption in circadian cycles
caused by flying across time zones. Melatonin is a
proven cure for jet lag. By taking melatonin, you can
"reset" your body clock so that you quickly adjust to
the time change.

Our recommendation for jet lag is very straightfor-
ward: If you are taking a trip that involves travel
across time zones, take 3 to 5 mg of melatonin prior to
bedtime once you reach your new destination. Continue to take melatonin at bedtime for four nights until
your body clock is completely reset. If you find yourself awakening too early in your new destination, you
can take another 1 to 3 mg of melatonin to help yourself fall back to sleep. When you return home, readjust
your body clock by taking 3 to 5 mg of melatonin

before your normal bedtime, and do so until you have readjusted to the time change. Many people claim that by taking melatonin they experience none of the symptoms normally associated with crossing time zones.

> If you are already taking melatonin daily as a part of our age-reversal therapy, is it all right to take additional melatonin to cure jet lag? Yes. Just follow the same instructions listed above.

GIVING MELATONIN A HELPING HAND

Melatonin is a powerful tool in helping to slow down the aging process, extend life, and maintain health. We do not want to leave you with the impression, however, that if you will only pop a melatonin capsule now and then you can neglect or abuse your body with impunity. It's not so simple. Melatonin can only keep you youthful and healthy if you let it.

In order to maintain the health of your pineal gland, your body's aging clock, you still need to maintain a healthy lifestyle. Here is some simple advice on how to stay healthy, and how to preserve your natural supply of melatonin.

Maintain a Normal Sleep/Wake Cycle

Your body works best when you follow your natural sleep/wake rhythm. Melatonin is not the only hormone that is released in a cyclical fashion. Your body is programmed to release many different hormones at different times throughout the day and night. Maintaining a reasonably normal schedule will help your body function at peak capacity.

Try to go to sleep around the same time every night, and try to awaken at about the same time every morning. Taking melatonin at night before bedtime can help maintain normal sleep patterns even if you've had trouble doing so in the past. We are not suggesting that you can't have late nights out, or that you should never "sleep in" on weekends. What we are saying is that you cannot constantly deprive yourself of sleep or subject yourself to erratic schedules without disrupting your body's natural hormonal cycles.

Our point is that sleep is essential for good health; it has a restorative effect on both the body and the psyche. It is when you are asleep that your melatonin levels peak and melatonin is pumped throughout your bloodstream to perform its many tasks. Lack of sleep can exact a steep toll on general health. People who routinely miss sleep are more prone to illness, and studies show that they even die younger than those who get enough sleep. Sleep deprivation also appears to promote premature aging. One study suggests that there may even be a strong correlation between premature wrinkling of the skin and lack of sleep.

We also recommend that you avoid behavior that can interfere with your ability to sleep. Try to make your evenings restful. If you exercise (and we recommend that you do), cease your exercise more than two hours before you intend to go to sleep. Studies show that strenuous exercise at night can blunt the nighttime increase in blood melatonin levels. Exercising too close to bedtime disrupts your sleep and melatonin cycles. (Just in case you were wondering, sex does not fall into the category of prohibited "vigorous exercise" at bedtime.)

How much sleep is enough sleep? Most people require around seven to eight hours a night to function well. Of course, some of us require less and some require more. You have to be the judge of how much sleep is enough. If you find that you're groggy during the day, and prone to dozing off, these are signs that you need more sleep. (For a more detailed discussion of sleep and the role of melatonin in treating sleep disorders, see Chapter 12.)

Don't Smoke

We seriously doubt that anyone reading this book needs to be told that smoking is bad for their heart, their lungs, and just about every organ and cell in their body. With each cigarette you inhale, you are ingesting thousands of chemicals, many of which are demonstrably carcinogenic. What you probably didn't know is that smoking can also disrupt your natural melatonin cycle. Given what we know about melatonin's role in protecting against cancer, this is particularly worrisome. By smoking, you are not only exposing your body to dangerous carcinogens, but you are depriving it of proper levels of the body's own very potent anticancer weapon, melatonin.

Avoid Excessive Alcohol

At least one of us, Walter, who is Italian, enjoys a glass or two of wine with his evening meal. Moderate drinking is no problem, but excessive alcohol consumption can damage every organ in your body, including your brain, heart, and liver. Alcohol, especially before bedtime, can also disrupt your nighttime production of melatonin.

Alcohol can induce sleepiness in many people. That is why some people drink a nightcap before bedtime to lull themselves to sleep. However, many such people find that within a few hours after falling asleep, they wake up and can't fall back to sleep. This occurs because alcohol disrupts the nighttime melatonin peak. Our advice is to avoid alcohol shortly before bedtime. (If you're taking melatonin, you won't need it anyway.)

Avoid Medications That Interfere with Melatonin

Several commonly used medications can severely disrupt natural melatonin cycles. We feel that these medications should be avoided whenever possible, or used with caution.

Many people take nonsteroidal anti-inflammatory medications (NSAIDS) such as aspirin and ibuprofen. These medications are typically prescribed for common problems such as arthritis or other types of joint and muscle pain. Although these medications are generally safe and effective, some people complain that when they are on these medications their sleep patterns are disrupted. This is not surprising. Studies have shown that NSAIDS can disrupt the normal nighttime melatonin cycle. If you are taking any of these medications and are having difficulty sleeping, you might ask your doctor to prescribe an alternative.

Beta-blockers, which are used to treat high blood pressure and heart disease, are another class of drugs that have been shown to interfere with melatonin production. It is especially problematic to take beta-blockers in the evening because they will abrogate the night peak of melatonin completely. People with high blood pressure who are taking beta-blockers have lower blood levels of melatonin than people with high blood pressure who are given other drugs such as diuretics (commonly known as water pills). In the section of this book on heart disease (see Chapter 8), we showed how melatonin can help normalize blood pressure and prevent other forms of coronary artery disease. High blood pressure often strikes during middle age or later, at just the point when natural melatonin levels begin to decline. Thus it strikes us as counterproductive to use a drug for high blood pressure that interferes with melatonin. There are several excellent medications for high blood pressure that can be given instead of beta-blockers. Taking melatonin may also help reduce high blood pressure. If you're on a beta-blocker for high blood pressure, do not discontinue your medication! That can be very dangerous. Do, however, talk to your physician about other treatment options.

Maintain Normal Weight

It is well known that maintaining an animal on a low-calorie but nutritious diet can increase its life span. A low-calorie diet does not extend life span as dramatically as melatonin does, nor does it have the same rejuvenating effect. However, there is ample documentation that when fed less food, an animal will live longer than if it is permitted to eat whatever it wants.

We also know that one of the quickest ways to shorten an animal's life span is to fatten it up. Animals who are fed high-fat, high-calorie diets are more prone to develop cancer and heart disease. The same is true for people. Obesity can cut life short.

Obesity, which is defined as being about 20 percent over your ideal weight, is a virtual epidemic in the United States. As many as one out of three Americans are considered obese, and, on average, Americans weigh ten pounds more than they did just a decade ago. Obesity is dangerous for several reasons; it can increase our risk of developing many dangerous diseases, including heart disease, cancer, diabetes, and stroke. Studies have also shown that obese people do not cycle melatonin normally. Clearly, obesity has a negative effect on the pineal gland, the body's aging clock.

What we find particularly alarming is that obesity is occurring at younger and younger ages. More than 25 percent of all American children are obese and are destined to become obese adults. What parents don't realize is that when children are allowed to become obese, they are being programmed to become obese adults, and consequently are at risk of dying young. Not only are they disrupting their melatonin production, they are seriously interfering with the function of other glands that are involved in growth and reproduction.

Being obese during puberty can have particularly serious health consequences for later life. Back in the 1970s, Walter devised an experiment in which he maintained mice on a reduced calorie diet for the first six weeks after weaning. Mice enter puberty at about that time. Walter maintained other newborn mice on a normal-calorie diet. After the first six weeks, he placed the first group on a normal-calorie diet as well. Throughout the initial six-week diet period, there were significant hormonal differences in the two groups. The mice on the low-calorie diet were half the size of the control mice and looked and acted much younger. Later, when they were allowed to eat freely, these former dieters quickly caught up to the other mice in terms of weight. Interestingly, however, even when the dieting mice were allowed to eat normally, their hormone levels still remained quite different from those of the other mice. In fact, their levels of corticosteroids—hormones produced during periods of stress —were much lower. It is well known that high levels of corticosteroids, which are often found in older animals, including humans, can cause many problems, including damage to the portion of the brain that controls memory.

From this experiment, Walter deduced that the reason the animals maintained on a low-calorie diet live longer was because their brains had actually developed differently. This could only be due to a permanent change in the hypothalamus, which, through its control of the pituitary gland, regulates many activities, including hunger, thirst, and sexual development. Somehow, by reducing food intake, the hypothalamus was programmed to keep the body younger, not just for the duration of the diet, but for long afterward. And although he didn't know it back then, we now know that animals kept on a low-calorie diet have higher levels of melatonin than those who are fed normally.

We're not advising that you starve or underfeed your children. We are saying that you do them a serious disservice if you continually feed them high-fat, high-calorie, sugar-laden foods and beverages that will program their endocrine glands to forever crave extra calories. Fruits, vegetables, low-fat dairy products, and lean meat and fish are better food choices for children and adults, and they will help you maintain a more youthful state.

One of the miracles of melatonin is that the science underlying its vast and varied powers is so elegant and accessible. Happily, melatonin is also readily available, inexpensive, and very simple to use. Our advice is not difficult to follow, nor does it involve expensive drugs or therapies or costly equipment. It does not require any more expenditure of precious time than is required to go to your neighborhood health-food store or pharmacy to purchase a bottle of melatonin. Part of *The Melatonin Miracle* is its simplicity and the fact that the promise of a longer and healthier life is now within the reach of us all.

AFTERWORD

Toward a New Paradigm of Aging

The Melatonin Miracle may be the first book you've seen written on melatonin, but we are confident that it will not be the last. Although we now know a great deal about melatonin and its key role in controlling the body's aging clock, scientists have only begun to tap its power. The story of the melatonin miracle is only at its beginning.

We hope that *The Melatonin Miracle* will inspire readers with its life-affirming message, that they will be excited about what it means for their future, and, most importantly, that it will encourage a change in the way most of us, including physicians and the medical profession, view aging. As scientists and as the authors of this book, above all else we hope that our work will serve as a catalyst for change. We want to challenge outdated notions of what "aging" means, and with that, outdated notions of what constitutes proper care from the medical profession. We want both for our generation and those that succeed us, not just more out of life, but more life. We are speaking about not only an increase in the quantity, but also in the quality of our years.

Our aim has been to give you a new model of aging,

a model that keeps up with the new reality. The time has come to discard the stereotype of the weak, frail elder and replace it with an image of ourselves growing "young" in strong, healthy bodies, enjoying much the same psychic and physical vigor that we associate with our youth.

We have said that we regard aging as the ultimate disease and as such we do not view the downward spiral of physical and mental decline that is generally accepted as a natural part of growing older as either inevitable or as something that should be accepted with such complacency. That precipitous decline, normally marked by progressive breakdowns in various bodily systems, is not a necessary nor an inevitable part of growing older. The progressive breakdown in bodily systems that occurs in our older years, and which is what makes us so much more vulnerable to illness, can be forestalled. It is by treating the underlying disease, which is aging itself, that we can intervene and break the aging → disease → aging cycle. When we succeed at this, we prevent both a major cause, and a major effect of "aging." In other words, the most effective solution to aging, as it is with any disease, is prevention.

Accordingly, we hope to revolutionize most particularly one facet of the practice of medicine: the way physicians tend to view, and therefore the way they tend to treat, their patients from the middle years on. What is currently standard practice—even by the very best and most skilled physicians—is to apply what is in truth a double standard when it comes to treating older patients. Consider the following: If a physician were to run a blood test on a twenty-year-old male patient and found an elevated level of blood sugar, the physician would be concerned and would promptly prescribe a special diet, medication, and exercise. In short, the physician would immediately look to cure what was perceived to be a problem. Now take the exact same scenario, but the patient this time is a sixty-year-old male. Upon seeing the elevated level of blood sugar in this patient, most physicians would dismiss the condition as the inevitable result of the patient's "advanced years." In other words, in the case of the sixty-year-old the exact same condition would be regarded as "normal" that in a twenty-year-old would be deemed as abnormal and needing treatment.

We think this is wrong. High blood glucose levels are dangerous to people of all ages (the condition can cause diabetes, hardening of the arteries, heart attack, and stroke), yet only in the twenty-year-old would the condition be treated aggressively. To our minds, this means too often we are sitting back and waiting for disease to strike a person just because he (or she) is sixty, seventy, eighty, ninety years old, and to us that is the antithesis of good medicine. We reject the depressing and fatalistic approach of contemporary medicine in this respect, which is to assume that what is abnormal in a young person is normal in a person above a certain age.

We recognize and appreciate how difficult it is to shake free of long-held assumptions that become so firmly fixed in our minds that they are no longer questioned. After all, we had to free ourselves of many such assumptions or otherwise we would never have accomplished the research that led us to the discovery of the "aging clock" and the power of melatonin to reset that clock for longer, healthier life. Without the courage to question conventional thought we would not have opened our minds or our eyes to the results of that research, which offered also the basis for our melatonin replacement therapy: The key to our approach to staying young, even as we accumulate years, is to restore melatonin levels to the levels that they were in our twenties, when our adult melatonin levels were at their peak and when we typically enjoyed our best health. By doing this, we can keep our pineal function working as it did in our youth and with that we can keep all of our body systems strong.

Maintaining the strength and function of our body systems is the key to breaking the aging → disease → aging cycle. By keeping our body systems in a "youthful state," we can prevent the debility and illness that has come to typify the aging process. By taking melatonin, we can stave off disease and maintain the full function of all of our body systems. We can live longer, fuller, and most importantly, healthier lives unmarred in our later years by a deteriorating body and crippling diseases.

We hope that the work we have described here helps make the case for the fact that there is a different and better way to age. We also hope that our work will encourage more research to be done in this area.

Finally, our hope in writing *The Melatonin Miracle* is not only to share with the public what few outside the scientific community know of these exciting discoveries, but also to share with readers our optimistic view of what life can and should be. We want you to understand that "senescence," the downward spiral that is now the hallmark of aging, is not inevitable, and that aging is neither irresistible nor irreversible. It is possible to retain our strength, sexual vigor, and love of life for all of our decades.

The miracle of melatonin is not just that it can extend your life and preserve your health and vigor. The true miracle of melatonin is the wider impact that it will have on our generation and on generations to come. We are embarking on an adventure together. We are the first generation to have the power to prevent the disease and the debility that have come to typify "normal" aging. For the first time, we have the power to preserve our youthfulness and to stay vital and vigorous for our entire lives. For the first time, not only are we able to prevent the physical decline associated with aging, but we're actually able to slow down and even reverse the aging process itself. This is truly the melatonin miracle.

Walter Pierpaoli, M.D., Ph.D.
William Regelson, M.D.
August 1995

Pineal Control of Aging: Effect of Melatonin and Pineal Grafting on Aging Mice

Walter Pierpaoli* and William Regelson†

ABSTRACT Dark-cycle, night administration of the pineal hormone melatonin in drinking water to aging mice (15 months of age) prolongs survival of BALB/c females from 23.8 to 28.1 months and preserves aspects of their youthful state. Similar results were seen in New Zealand Black females beginning at 5 months and C57BL/6 males beginning at 19 months. As melatonin is produced in circa-

* Biancalana-Masera Foundation for the Aged (Convention I.N.R.C.A. and University of Ancona), Neuroimmunomodulation Laboratory, via Birarelli 8, 60121 Ancona, Italy.
† Medical College of Virginia, Virginia Commonwealth University, Box 273, Richmond, VA 23298.

Communicated by Samuel M. McCann, July 29, 1993 (received for review January 15, 1992).

Abbreviations: NZB, New Zealand Black: DTH, delayed-type hypersensitivity.

dian fashion from the pineal, we grafted pineals from young 3- to 4-month-old donors into the thymus of 20-month-old syngeneic C57BL/6 male recipients, and a 12% increase in survival was induced. Prolongation of survival was also seen on pineal transplant to the thymus in C57BL/6, BALB/cJ, and hybrid female mice at 16, 19, and 22 months. In all studies, the endogenous pineal of grafted mice was left *in situ*. Pineal grafted aged mice display a remarkable maintenance of thymic structure and cellularity. Preservation of T-cell-mediated function, despite age, as measured by response to oxazolone is seen. Other evidence suggests that melatonin and/or pineal-related factors could produce their effects through an influence on thyroid function. These data indicate that pineal influences have a place in the physiologic regulation of aging.

The pineal hormone melatonin is secreted in all mammals during the dark phase of the circadian cycle (1), but, even more importantly, there are indications that it is a key regulator of aging and senescence (2, 3). The role of melatonin in controlling sexual maturity, sexual cycling, cancer, stress, and the immune response makes it likely that the pineal may be a factor in the syndrome of aging (4–6). With this in mind, we have administered exogenous melatonin in the drinking water of mice during a fixed circadian dark cycle—i.e., when melatonin is normally produced—in order to ascertain its influence on patterns of survival.

In addition, as the pineal gland is the prime source of melatonin, we transplanted the pineal gland from young to syngeneic histocompatible older recipients. We have utilized the thymus as the graft recipient site inasmuch as the thymus and the pineal gland share a common adrenergic innervation via the superior cervical ganglion (7, 8). This common innervation is of importance as melatonin synthesis is inhibited by pharmacologic sympathetic blockade, which also modulates the immune response

Appendix 1

(9). Moreover, the pineal morphologically contains lymphocytes and it has been likened in its embryologic developmental origin to the thymus (10).

In our studies, exogenous nocturnal circadian administration of melatonin or engraftment of young homologous (3–4 months) pineals to old (18–22 months) syngeneic mice adjacent to the thymus, leaving the recipient's pineal *in situ,* resulted in a significant enhancement of survival independent of significant weight loss. These results suggest that the pineal may act as an endogenous clock governing aging.

MATERIALS AND METHODS

Melatonin Administration. Mice were fed ad libitum using NAFAG pellets (Gossau, Switzerland) and housed 4–10 to a cage in air-conditioned quarters at 22°C. Light exposure was controlled by a fixed timer that governs a standard fluorescent fixture (Philips TLD 36W/84). Melatonin, solubilized in ethanol, was given in the drinking water during a fixed darkness cycle from 6 p.m. to 8:30 a.m. (10 µg/ml of tap water, 0.01% ethanol). The control (only ethanol) and melatonin-containing water bottles were removed from 8:30 a.m. to 6 p.m. No drinking water was given during that period. The mice were individually weighed at intervals to determine whether the effects seen were related to dietary intake.

Pineal Grafting. In young-to-old, pineal-to-thymus grafting, the "young" pineals were obtained from 3- to 4-month-old, postpubertal mice. Syngeneic recipients were groups of "aging" mice. The recipient mice were uniform as to sex and age, housed 3–7 per cage. They were prepared for surgery and studied in groups, as indicated in Tables 1 and 2. Weight changes of control and pineal-transplanted animals were recorded monthly.

Donor mice were killed by cervical dislocation and the skull fragment to which the pineal gland adheres was removed and immersed in cooled TC 199 medium containing penicillin and streptomycin. The pineal was carefully separated with fine scissors and removed *in situ* within its original supporting membranes, maintenance of which aids graft vascularization.

Grafts recipients were anesthetized by i.p. injection of a barbiturate (Vetanarcol; Veterinaria, Zurich). Thereafter, the shaven chest was prepped with 70% ethanol and a 5- to 8-mm-long midline skin incision was made commencing just below the neck. A 2- to 3-mm length of the thorax was opened and the mediastinal tissue was exposed and the native thymus became available *in situ* by exerting moderate pressure on the abdomen. A single donor pineal gland was positioned on the tip of a hollow needle and introduced into the needle by gentle aspiration. The pineal graft was injected slowly into the right or left lobe of the thymus with rotation of the needle. Occasionally at surgery, when a successful transplantation of the pineal was in doubt, a second pineal gland was used. The sternum, muscles, and skin were then sutured and a protective plastic film (Nobecutan, Bofors, Sweden) was sprayed on the wound. In a few instances the operation led to immediate death of the mice due to hemorrhage or pneumothorax. Control groups were similarly transplanted into the thymus with a pineal-size matched fragment from the donor brain cortex.

Immune response was measured by the delayed-type hypersensitivity (DTH) response to oxazolone (2). Statistics used equal variance t test for unpaired normal samples (two tailed).

Light Microscopy. Serial sections (5 μm) of thymic pineal grafts and thyroids were obtained from 21-month-old BALB/c female mice at sacrifice 3 months after pineal grafting in 5–10 animals from control and treated groups. The sections were stained with hematoxylin/eosin and examined microscopically in blinded fashion without knowledge of which experimental group they belonged to.

Appendix 1

RESULTS

Oral Administration of Melatonin. Fig. 1 depicts a survival comparison between normal controls and melatonin-treated BALB/c female mice. The average survival of controls was 715 days vs. 843 days for melatonin-treated mice. In the controls (Fig. 1) median survival was 23.8 months, whereas the median melatonin-treated survival was 28.1 months, with an absolute upper limit of survival on melatonin administration of 29.4 months as compared to 27.2 months for controls. Equal variance t test for unpaired normal samples treated vs. controls showed $P < 0.001$. There were no significant differences in weight between the two groups at any time.

Fig. 2 shows prolongation of life when NZB mice were given melatonin in the drinking water, daily, at night, with no effect seen when melatonin was given during daylight hours. Using log-rank values comparing control with night-administered melatonin showed a P value of 0.059. The common causes of death in all melatonin-treated or control NZB mice were autoimmune hemolytic anemia, nephrosclerosis, and development of a systemic or localized type A or B reticulum cell neoplasia, which characterizes end-stage disease in these aging mice.

Fig. 3 shows results of melatonin treatment, starting at 19 months of age in C57BL/6 male mice. Melatonin in drinking water prolonged the absolute duration of life by up to 6 months when compared to untreated controls. The average weight changes of the melatonin-treated mice as compared with controls were not a factor in survival.

Implantation of a Pineal from Young Donors into the Thymus of Aging Recipients. Table 1 shows the pattern of survival in pineal-implanted C57BL/6, BALB/c × C57BL/6 hybrids, and BALB/c females, pineal engrafted at 16, 19, and 22 months, respectively. All untreated con-

Appendix 1

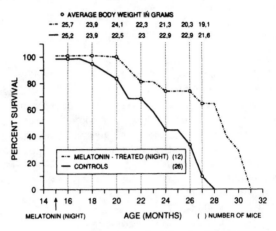

FIGURE 1. *Aging postponement and/or life prolongation in BALB/c female mice consequent to night administration of melatonin.*

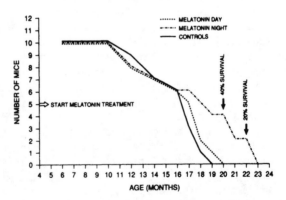

FIGURE 2. *Survival in New Zealand Black (NZB) female mice given melatonin in drinking water. Day versus night. [Reprinted with permission from ref. 2 (copyright New York Academy of Sciences).]*

Appendix 1

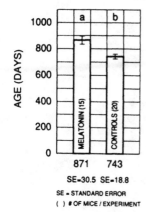

FIGURE 3. *Survival in C57BL/6 male mice consequent to melatonin, during dark cycle, beginning at 19 months when mice show onset of age-related death. [Reprinted (with modification) with permission from ref. 2 (copyright New York Academy of Sciences).]*

trols were dead at 26 months, whereas several pineal/ thymus-transplanted animals were still alive at 31 months, and there was a significant prolongation of life in all three grafted groups. As seen in Table 1, P values ranged from < 0.01 to < 0.05 in comparing control vs. pineal-transplanted groups, and weight loss was not a factor.

The effect of pineal engraftment into the thymus (Fig. 4) showed prolonged survival in the 20-month-old C57BL/6 male mice grafted with a pineal from 3-month-old syngeneic donors. In this study, although the significant difference between pineal-grafted and controls resulted in only a 12% enhancement of survival, the absolute range of survival in the treated animals is > 810 days, with a single animal (not counted in final evaluation) surviving 1035 days as compared to 747 days for control animals. The standard error is indicated in Fig. 4. Body weight changes did not contribute to survival between pineal-grafted and control groups. No life-prolonging effect was seen in the control group implanted into the thymus with a pineal-size fragment of brain cortex.

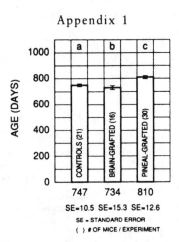

FIGURE 4. *Survival following pineal transplantation into 20-month-old C57BL/6 male recipients from 3-month-old donors.*

These results fully confirmed our observations in C57BL/6, BALB/cJ, and hybrid females as can be seen in Table 1. Most important, pineal engraftment was performed in different aged groups: 16-, 19-, and 22-month-old mice. The engrafted mice, in some cases, lived for an increased lifespan of 4–6 months, with a median of 4.2, 4.5, and over 6.5 months longer than controls (Table 1). The effect of pineal engraftment from young to old resulted in a 17%, 21%, and 27% increase in absolute survival ($P < 0.01$ or < 0.05, Table 1).

Fig. 5 shows the typical morphology of a residual pineal gland from a 3-month-old donor mouse grafted to the thymus of an 18-month-old recipient, at 3 months after transplantation. Donor and recipient were inbred, histo-compatible BALB/cJ mice. Identical results were seen in grafting the pineal to 6-month-old and 20-month-old recipients.

As can be seen, typical normal and viable clusters of pinealocytes are still assembled within the intact, transplanted pineal gland, which closely maintains its original

Appendix 1

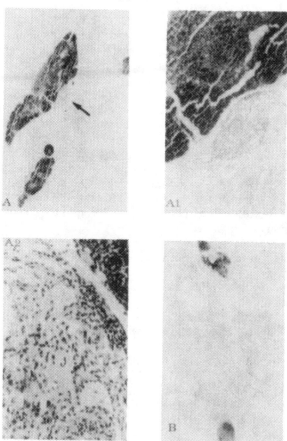

FIGURE 5. *Viable pineal gland in the thymus of a 21-month-old BALB/c female mouse at 3 months after grafting. (A) The arrow indicates the site of implantation, close to a thymic lobe, whose cellularity and structure are largely maintained. (A1) Notice the remarkable maintenance of a typical thymic cortex, with densely packed thymocytes. (A2) Clusters of viable pinealocytes can be seen in the grafted pineal. (B) Residual thymic rudiment of a 21-month-old BALB/c female mouse. Notice the presence of two atrophic small lymph nodes. (Hematoxylin/eosin; A and B, ×20; A1, ×70; A2, ×260.)*

267

structure. Perhaps the most remarkable finding was that in all sacrificed animals at advanced age (21 months), the thymic structure of the pineal-grafted mice is still maintained (Fig. 5A and A1), whereas in control samples the thymus contained no residual thymic lymphocytes (Fig. 5B).

As illustrated in Table 2, melatonin treatment and pineal grafting resulted in a significant maintenance of a vigorous immunological response expressing cell-mediated transplantation immunity, as measured by DTH response to oxazolone. Significance is indicated in the legend to Table 2, where the immune reactivity, present in pineal-grafted mice as compared to controls, confirmed the histologic observation of repopulation of the thymus seen in pineal-grafted mice (Fig. 5).

Recent observations on thyroid function in melatonin-treated mice (2) prompted us to examine thyroid morphology in pineal-grafted senescent mice. Light microscopy of the thyroid gland of pineal-grafted and control aging mice in our "blinded" histologic study showed a very remarkable maintenance of a youthful thyroid morphology, as compared to control (Fig. 6).

DISCUSSION

If aging is a neuroendocrine programmed event, the role of the pineal in governing circadian and circannual rhythms, pubertal development, and seasonal sexual cycling suggests that it may have a place in the programming or prevention of senescence (1–4). In support of this there is an age-related decrease in melatonin values in the pineal itself and in the circulating levels of melatonin (11). Clinically, Touitou *et al.* (12) and others (2) have found that clinical levels of plasma melatonin in elderly patients show a significant decline.

Melatonin treatment in C57BL/6 male mice beginning at 19 months prolonged absolute duration of survival by

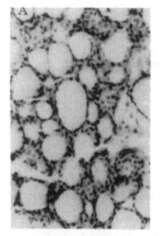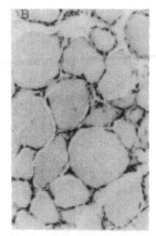

FIGURE 6. *Maintenance of juvenile structure and function in the thyroid gland of aging BALB/c mice grafted into the thymus with a pineal gland from young donors. (A) Pineal-grafted: Notice normal cellular and follicle size and structure. (B) Control: Notice flattened epithelium and distended follicles as a manifestation of hypofunction. (Hematoxylin/eosin; × 130.)*

6 months. Similar tests were seen in BALB/c female mice and in NZB mice, with melatonin treatment onset at 15 and at 5 months, respectively. These NZB female treated mice given melatonin during the dark cycle showed a 20% increase in survival at 22 months, with all controls dead at 19 months.

Most important, when youthful pineals were engrafted into aging 16-, 19-, and 22-month-old mice, the engrafted mice, in some cases, lived for an increased lifespan of 4 to > 6 months, with a median of 4.2, 4.5, and over 6.5 months longer than controls (Table 1). The effect of pineal engraftment from young to old resulted in a 17%, 21%, and 27% increase in absolute survival. This is further confirmed by a 12% increase in absolute survival on pineal to thymus engraftment from young mice to 20-month-old C57BL/6 mice (Fig. 4). In these studies,

Table 1. Implantation of a pineal gland from young 3- to 4-month-old donors into the thymus of old aging, strain- and sex-matched mice postpones aging and/or prolongs the life of the pineal-implanted recipients

Group	Strain and treatment	Age at implant or sham-operated, months	No.	No. of surviving mice (months of age)																
				17	18	19	20	21	22	23	24	25	26	27	28	29	30	31	32	33
A	Implanted C57BL/6	16	7	7	7	7	7	7	6	6	5	4	3	3	2	1	1	1	0	
B	Control C57BL/6	16	7	6	6	6	4	4	2	1	1	0	0	0	0	0	0	0		
C	Implanted hybrids*	19	5	—	—	—	5	5	5	5	5	5	5	5	5	5	4	3	2	1
D	Control hybrids	19	6	—	—	—	6	6	4	3	2	1	0	0	0	0	0			
E	Implanted BALB/cJ	22	3	—	—	—	—	—	—	3	3	3	3	3	3	3	1	1	0	
F	Control BALB/cJ	22	5	—	—	—	—	—	—	5	5	2	2	0	0	0	0			

*C57BL/6 × BALB/cJ female hybrids. All donor and recipient mice used were inbred females. For details on the method and technique, see text. Data have been published in ref. 2. A vs. B: $P < 0.05$ (Mann–Whitney U test). C vs. D: $P < 0.01$ (Mann–Whitney U test). E vs. F: $P < 0.05$ (Mann–Whitney U test).

Table 2. Dark cycle treatment with melatonin or transplantation of pineal glands from young donors maintains DTH response and retards aging in old mice

Group	Treatment	Strain	Sex	No.	Age, months	Melatonin, months of treatment	DTH response to oxazolone[a] Before challenge	After challenge	Survival, days
A	Untreated	BALB/cJ	♀	9	26	—	28.25 ± 4.57	31.62 ± 7.11 (+12%)[b]	716 ± 101
B	Melatonin	BALB/cJ	♀	15	26	10	25.69 ± 1.96	31.06 ± 4.22 (+21%)[c]	843 ± 39 (+18%)[j]
C	Pineal[d]	BALB/cJ	♀	6	26	—	26.00 ± 3.60	33.67 ± 3.06 (+30%)[e]	902 ± 35 (+26%)[i]
D	Untreated	C57BL/6	♀	22	25	—	24.38 ± 2.14	29.62 ± 3.11 (+22%)[f]	773 ± 121
E	Melatonin	C57BL/6	♀	22	25	7	23.26 ± 1.06	29.93 ± 3.76 (+29%)[g]	826 ± 110 (+7%)[k]
F	Untreated	C57BL/6	♂	8	23	—	32.44 ± 4.52	34.72 ± 3.21 (+7%)[b]	743 ± 84
G	Melatonin	C57BL/6	♂	10	23	7	27.75 ± 0.99	33.33 ± 4.00 (+20%)[h]	871 ± 118 (+17%)[l]

Analysis of variance: after challenge compared with before challenge (see *Materials and Methods* and *Results*). [a]Data are presented as mean ± SD. [b]Not significant (NS). [c]$P < 0.005$. [d]Five months after implantation into the thymus of a pineal from a young, 3-month-old donor. [e]$P < 0.001$. [f]$P < 0.0001$. [g]$P < 0.005$. Statistics of survival (days, Mann–Whitney U test): [i]$P < 0.05$, C vs. A; [j]$P < 0.001$, B vs. A; [k]NS, E vs. D; [l]$P < 0.001$, G vs. F.

melatonin-treated and pineal to thymus-grafted mice, despite the advanced age of recipients, show preservation of T-cell-mediated immune function as measured by the DTH response to oxazolone (Table 2).

In the pineal-grafted animals, survival data are reinforced by the apparent juvenile morphologic state of the thymus and thyroid and the immune status of recipients despite their age (Figs. 5 and 6). The maintenance of thymic function is not surprising as melatonin and the pineal are known to enhance the immune response 9, 10, 13–18). This may well delay the appearance of tumors (19) and autoimmune disease (20) as factors in age-related pathology.

Melatonin has been shown to block ovulation and is now being evaluated as a clinical contraceptive (21). In that regard, the pineal adapts the internal neuroendocrine environment to changes in external variables that can involve not only exposure to light but also humidity, magnetism, temperature, antigens, pheromones, hunger, sexual drive, fear, and distress (1, 2, 4, 22). Pineal function may have a complementary modulating role against stress-mediated corticosteroid action (2–3, 4, 6, 14–16, 23–28). Russian data suggests that a pineal polypeptide may reduce sensitivity to dexamethasone (26). Anisimov *et al.* (29) have found a pineal peptide that delays aging, which may be a factor in preventing oncogenesis (30).

Apart from melatonin and as yet undefined pineal peptides (26, 29, 30), the pineal also contains thyrotropin-releasing hormone (TRH) (31, 32) and modulates the 5′ thyroid deiodinase (33). TRH and melatonin can block steroid- or stress-related thymic involution (9, 16, 34, 35) and restore immunocompetence in nude (athymic) mice (16). TRH and melatonin have receptors in the preoptic hypothalamic areas of the brain important to thyroid and thymus regulation (22, 24, 34, 35).

The pineal graft may act directly on its thymic neighbor via melatonin or possibly via other pineal hormones that

Appendix 1

diffuse into the thymus. The grafted pineal may receive sympathetic fibers from the superior cervical ganglion, which normally innervates the thymus, and thus may have a normal pattern of nocturnal melatonin release that acts on the thymus to rejuvenate the gland.

Whatever the mechanism, maintenance of immune responsiveness follows youthful pineal engraftment, and thymic and thyroid morphologic restoration occurs at a time when the normal involution of age is demonstrable. Our exogenous use of circadian melatonin and pineal engraftment of young pineals to the site of the thymus in aged mice suggests that there may be a firm relationship between the pineal, its products, and the thymus, providing a homeostatic control mechanism of significance for aging and survival.

We thank Ms. Monica Bacciarini Rossi for technical help and Dr. Keith Dixon and Mr. Kurt Rotach for the statistical studies. We are indebted to Dr. Richard Cutler (National Institute on Aging, Baltimore) for contributing mice used in the pineal transplant experiments. The mice used in all other experiments were a generous gift from CIBA-Geigy (Animal Breeding Center, Sisseln, Switzerland). We are grateful to the late Dr. Maurice Landy (La Jolla, CA) for editorial help. Also, the help of Dr. Ennio Pedrinis (Istituto Cantonale di Patologia, Locarno, Switzerland) for analysis of light microscopy and the photographs of Figs. 5 and 6 is gratefully acknowledged. We also acknowledge the cooperation of the *Annals of the New York Academy of Sciences* in permitting us to publish Figs. 2 and 3 and Table 1 from our previous work (2).

1. Hastings, M. H., Vance, G. & Maywood, E. (1989) *Experientia* **45**, 903–1008.
2. Pierpaoli, W., Dall'Ara, A., Pedrinis, E. & Regelson, W. (1991) *Ann. N.Y. Acad. Sci.* **621**, 291–313.
3. Pierpaoli, W. (1991) *Aging* **3**, 99–101.

Appendix 1

4. Reiter, R. J., Craft, C. M. & Johnson, J. E. (1981) *Endocrinology* **109**, 1205–1207.

5. Hoffmann, K., Illnerova, H. & Vaneck, I. (1985) *Neurosci. Lett.* **56**, 39–43.

6. Thomas, D. R. & Miles, A. (1989) *Bio. Psychol.* **25**, 365–367.

7. Bulloch, K. (1985) in *Neural Modulation of Immunity*, eds. Guillemin, R., Cohn, M. & Melnechuk, T. (Raven, New York), pp. 111–141.

8. Erlich, S. S. & Apuzzo, M. L. J. (1985) *Neurosurgery* **63**, 321–341.

9. Maestroni, G. J. M., Conti, A. & Pierpaoli, W. (1986) *J. Neuroimmunol.* **13**, 19–30.

10. Vede, T., Ishi, Y. & Matsume, A. (1981) *Anat. Rec.* **199**, 239–247.

11. Trentini, G. B., Genazzani, A. R., Criscuolo, M., Petraglia, F., De Gaetani, C., Ficarra, G., Bidzinska, B., Migaldi, M. & Genazzani, A. D. (1992) *Neuroendocrinology* **56**, 364–370.

12. Touitou, Y., Feure-Montagne, M. & Prouse, J. (1985) *Acta Endocrinol.* **108**, 135–144.

13. Pierpaoli, W. & Sorkin, E. (1972) *Nature New Biol.* **238**, 282–285.

14. Pierpaoli, W. & Besedovsky, H. O. (1975) *Clin. Exp. Immunol.* **20**, 323–328.

15. Pierpaoli, W. (1981) in *Psychoneuroimmunology*, ed. Ader, R. (Academic, New York). pp. 575–606.

16. Pierpaoli, W. & Yi, C. X. (1990) *J. Neuroimmunol.* **37**, 99–110.

17. del Gorbo, V., Cibri, V. & Villani, N. (1989) *Int. J. Immunol.* **11**, 567–573.

18. Fraschini, F., Scaglione, F. & Franco, P. (1990) *Acta Oncol.* **29**, 775–776.

19. Regelson, W. & Pierpaoli, W. (1987) *Cancer Invest.* **5**, 379–385.

20. Hansson, I., Holmdahl, R. & Mattsson, R. (1990) *J. Neuroimmunol.* **27**, 79–84.

Appendix 1

21. Voordouw, B. C., Euser, R., Verdonk, R. G., Alberda, B. T., De Jong, F. H., Drogendijk, A. C., Fauser, B. J. M. & Cohen, M. (1992) *J. Clin. Endocrinol. Metab.* **74,** 108–117.

22. Rebuffat, P., Mazzocchi, G. & Stachowiak, A. (1988) *Exp. Clin. Endocrinol.* **91,** 59–64.

23. Wurtman, R. J., Alschule, M. D. & Holmgren, U. (1959) *Am. J. Physiol.* **197,** 59–64.

24. Demisch, L., Demisch, J. & Nikelsen. T. (1988) *J. Pineal Res.* **5,** 317–322.

25. Sharma, M., Palacois-Bois, J. & Schwartz, G. (1989) *Biol. Psychol.* **25,** 305–319.

26. Golikov, P. P. (1973) *Endocrinology* **19,** 100–102.

27. Khan, R., Kaya, S. & Potgieter, B. (1990) *Experientia* **46,** 860–862.

28. Yuwiler, A. (1985) *J. Neurochem.* **44,** 1185–1193.

29. Anisimov, V. N., Loktionov, A. S. & Khavinson, V. (1989) *Mech. Ageing Dev.* **49,** 1185–1193.

30. Bartsch, H., Bartsch, C., Simon, W. E., Flehmig, B., Ebels, I. & Lippert, T. H. (1992) *Oncology* **49,** 27–30.

31. Lew, G. M. (1989) *Histochemistry* **91,** 43–46.

32. Vriend, J. (1978) *Med. Hypothesis* **4,** 376–387.

33. Guerrero, J. M. & Reiter, R. J. (1992) *Int. J. Biochem.* **24,** 1513–1523.

34. Lesnikov, V. A., Dall'Ara, A., Korneva, E. A. & Pierpaoli, W. (1992) *Int. J. Neurosci.* **62,** 741–753.

35. Ruczas, C. (1988) in *Fundamental Clinics in Pineal Research,* eds. Trentini, G. P., DeGaetani, C. & Pevet, P. (Raven, New York), pp. 257–270.

Pineal Cross-Transplantation (Old-to-Young and Vice Versa) as Evidence for an Endogenous "Aging Clock"

Vladimir A. Lesnikov* and Walter Pierpaoli†

We have shown that both exogenous, chronic circadian (night) administration of the pineal neurohormone melatonin (N-acetyl-5-methoxytryptamine) to old mice or grafting of the entire pineal gland from young donors into the thymus of aging mice delays aging and prolongs a state of juvenile, disease-free life.[1-4] However, in both models used, some aspects were as yet amenable to criticism, which required clarification. In fact, in those time-

* Present address: R/D Haemoderivitaves, SCLAVO SpA, Via Fiorentina, 1, 53100 Siena, Italy.
† Novera H. Spector Neuroimmunomodulation Laboratory, Biancalana-Masera Foundation for the Aged, Via Birarelli, 8, 60121 Ancona, Italy. Requests for reprints should be addressed to: Institute of Experimental Medicine, Russian Academy of Medical Science, St. Petersburg, Russia.

Appendix 2

consuming experiments one could not completely dis-
criminate the positive effects of chronic melatonin administration or pineal grafting from changes related to
different food intake, drinking habits, chronic stimulation
of the thymus, etc., which would not allow drawing con-
clusions about a real life-prolonging effect of the treatment when compared with the control groups.

We devised experiments which would permit evaluat-
ing beyond any possible doubt whether the life-
prolonging or aging-delaying effects observed were due
to the intrinsic properties of the pineal and not to nonspecific chronic factors, in that the mice used were themselves controls, donors and at the same time recipients of
an "old" or of a "young" pineal gland.

A few years ago we initiated a new series of long-term
experiments with a genetically pure, inbred strain of
mice, namely the BALB/cJ, in which the entire pineal
gland adhering to the bone fragment of the skull was removed simultaneously from the skull of young-adult (3–
4-month-old) or old (18-month-old) mice of the same
inbred strain and sex, and in which the size- and shape-
matched skull fragment with the "young" or the "old"
pineals were adapted to the skull of the young or old
recipient. This operation is described in Figure 1.

PINEAL CROSS-TRANSPLANTATION

Groups of female, young-adult (3–4-month-old) and old
aging (18-month-old) BALB/cJ mice maintained in our
animal rooms were used. They were kept at 22°C and had
free access to food pellets and tap water. Lighting of the
rooms was 7 a.m. light-on and 7 p.m. light-off. The animals were anesthetized with the barbiturate hexenal (200
mg/Kg). The upper part of the skull was accurately
shaven and the operation field was treated and disin-
fected with 70 percent ethanol, trying to avoid an irrita-
tion to the eyes. The head skin was cut sagittally along

Appendix 2

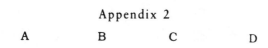

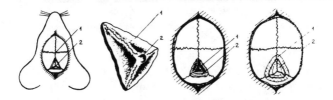

FIGURE 1. *Pineal cross-transplantation: sequential steps of the operation. (A) Operation field on the mouse head. The bone-pineal graft* (triangle) *is outlined by a double line. 1: bregma; 2: lambda. (B) Bone-pineal graft. 1: skull fragment inside the head bone; 2: pineal gland. (C) Cranial window in the recipient mouse. 1: cortex; 2: cerebellum. (D) Donor bone-pineal graft fitted to the recipient mouse. 1: cement; 2: bone-pineal graft fitted to the recipient mouse.*

the midline for 10–12 mm, and the aponeurosis and other soft tissues were removed from this part of the skull (see Fig. 1A). The surface of the bone was rinsed with 5 percent H_2O_2 and dried with 70 percent ethanol, in order to visualize the fissures of the calvarium. In order to fasten the mouse and to turn its head in a proper operational position, an original stereotaxical instrument developed at the Institute of Experimental Medicine, St. Petersburg, Russia, was used.[5,6]

A triangle-shaped skull fragment located at the intersection of the sagittal and occipital fissures (Fig.1A) was cut with the help of a dental drilling machine, trying not to produce any lesion to the underlying cortex and cerebellum. The next steps of the operation were carried out with the help of a dissection microscope. After turning the animal's head around its midline horizontal axis, the skull fragment, including its adherent pineal gland in its membranes and ligaments was removed. Bleeding from

279

the brain venous sinuses was stopped by repeated rinsing with saline and absorption with tissue pads until spontaneous cessation. The pineal ligaments connected with dura mater and forming the brain sinuses were cut with fine scissors and the skull fragment together with the adherent pineal gland was removed and kept in ice-cooled medium TC 199 (no serum added). It is also possible to use the same procedure to obtain skull fragments with epiphyses in their original position from mice which have been sacrificed as donors of an intact pineal gland. In all cases the bone-pineal graft must be examined microscopically to ensure that the pineal gland is in its original position and undamaged (Fig. 1B).

The pineal gland in its original position from the donor-recipient mouse is then positioned in the corresponding and size-matched, appropriate recipient-donor cranial window and the adapted skull fragment is glued with cement (polymer BF-6, Fig. 1C and D). After drying, the scalp skin is sutured with silk stitches and the sealed operation field is sprayed with antibiotic powder. The duration of one intervention of cross-transplantation between an old and a young mouse is between one and a half and two hours. Sham-operated mice undergo the same procedure, but the mouse is grafted again with its own skull fragment and pineal gland.

In the evaluation of the effects produced by pineal cross-transplantation between young and old mice, a noninvasive approach was chosen in order to assess the existence of a pineal "aging clock." We examined only body weights, physical conditions and the life span of the pineal, cross-grafted mice. A first series of mice (5 in each group) was cross-grafted in April 1990 and a second series in November 1991. Table 1 shows the results of both experiments. A remarkable acceleration of aging and death was seen in the young mice grafted with an "old" pineal, while a very significant delay of aging and death was observed in the old mice grafted with a

Appendix 2

TABLE 1. Pineal Gland, Young-to-Old and Old-to-Young Cross-Transplantation in BALB/cJ Female Mice Results in Prolongation or Abbreviation of Their Life Span under Conventional Laboratory Conditions[a]

Group	No.	Treatment	Survival (Days ± SE)[*]
A	30	sham-operated	719 ± 32
B	10	"young" pineal into old mice	1021 ± 56[***]
C	10	"old" pineal into young mice	510 ± 36[**]

[a] Young (4-month-old) and old (18-month-old) female inbred BALB/c mice were used simultaneously both as donors and as recipients of an intact pineal gland. The mice were left undisturbed after ear-marking as long as they lived. Their body weight was taken monthly. Results are of two identical experiments in the course of three years.

[*] Standard error; [**] C vs A, $p < 0.01$; [***] B vs A, $p < 0.002$. For statistical analysis the Student t test was used.

"young" pineal gland. At one year after the pineal cross-grafting, no evidence of age difference consequent to physical attrition and decay could be observed between the younger and the older mice (Fig. 2). A progressive increase of body weight was measured in the older mice grafted with a "young" pineal while the body weight of the younger mice grafted with an "old" pineal became progressively similar or identical to those of the older mice at about one year after pineal cross-grafting. In both cases death was preceded by a rapid loss of weight. This weight decrease was more marked in the younger mice grafted with an "old" pineal gland. Without exception, young-to-old or old-to-young pineal grafting respectively delayed or accelerated aging of a good one-third (6 months), which is about one-fourth the life duration of BALB/cJ mice in our animal rooms.[4] These results largely surpass the life prolongation and/or aging-delaying effects obtained with melatonin administration and/or pineal grafting into the thymus.[1-4] They clearly point to a distinctive and central role of the pineal gland in the initiation and progression of aging. This model deserves repetition and extension aimed at elucidating the mechanism by which the "aging clock" in the pineal scans the time of life and death.[7]

281

Appendix 2

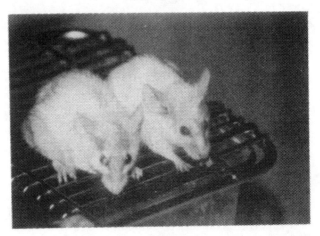

FIGURE 2. *Pineal cross-transplantation: effects on somatic conditions. The illustration shows two female inbred BALB/c mice at one year after pineal cross-grafting. The mouse on the* left *side was grafted at 540 days of age with the pineal gland from a 110-day-old donor. This mouse lived 1061 days. The mouse on the* right *side was grafted at 110 days of age with the pineal gland from the 540-day-old donor-recipient (on the* left *side of the picture). This younger mouse lived only 476 days. At one year after pineal cross-grafting no difference of somatic conditions (fur, posture, skin, weight) can be observed between the "old" and the "young" mouse.*

SUMMARY

Circadian (night), chronic administration of melatonin and young-to-old pineal grafting into the thymus have provided evidence for the existence of an endogenous, primary and central "aging clock" in the pineal gland. The new model described here serves to definitely demonstrate that the replacement of the pineal gland of an old mouse with the pineal from a young, syngeneic donor mouse remarkably prolongs its life and, conversely, the "old" pineal transplanted into a younger mouse will considerably shorten its life span. Pineal cross-transplantation thus provides clear-cut evidence for the central role of the pineal gland in the initiation and progression of senescence. It offers a novel basis for interventions in the aging process.

REFERENCES

1. Pierpaoli, W., & G. Maestroni. 1987. Melatonin: a principal neuroimmunoregulatory and anti-stress hormone. Its anti-aging effects. *Immunol. Lett.* **16:** 355–362.
2. Pierpaoli, W., & C-X. Yi. 1990. The involvement of pineal gland and melatonin in immunity and aging. I. Thymus-mediated, immunoreconstituting and antiviral activity of thyrotropin releasing hormone. *J. Neuroimmunol.* **27:** 99–109.
3. Pierpaoli, W., A. Dall 'Ara, E. Pedrinis *et al.* 1991. The pineal control of aging: the effects of melatonin and pineal grafting on the survival of older mice. In *Physiological Senescence and Its Postponement: Theoretical Approaches and Rational Interventions.* W. Pierpaoli & N. Fabris, eds. Ann. N.Y. Acad. Sci. **621:** 291–313.
4. Pierpaoli, W., & W. Regelson. 1994. Pineal control of aging: effect of melatonin and pineal grafting on aging mice. *Proc. Natl. Acad. Sci. USA* **94:** 787–791.
5. Kiyko, V. V., & V. A. Lesnikov. Stereotaxis Apparatus for Rodents. Certificate of Invention. Application No. 4713811/14. Filed at the USSR State Committee for Inventions and Discoveries, May 26, 1989.
6. Lesnikov, V. A., E. A. Korneva, A. DalL 'Ara *et al.* 1992. The involvement of pineal gland and melatonin in immunity and aging. II. Thyrotropin releasing hormone and melatonin forestall involution and promote reconstitution of the thymus in anterior hypothalamic

area (AHA)-lesioned mice. *Int. J. Neurosci.* **62:** 141–153.

7. Pierpaoli, W. The pineal aging clock. Evidence, models and an approach to aging-delaying strategies. In *Aging, Immunity and Infection.* D. C. Powers, J. E. Morley & R. M. Coe, eds. Springer Publishing Company. New York. In press.

SELECTED BIBLIOGRAPHY

Anisimov. V., Khavinson, K. H., and Morozov, V. G. "Twenty Years of Study on the Effects of Pineal Peptide Preparation: Epithalamin in Experimental Gerontology and Oncology." *Annals of the N.Y. Academy of Science* 719:483–93. 1994.

Arendt, J., Borbely, A. A., Franey C., and Wright, J. "The Effect of Chronic, Small Doses of Melatonin Given in the Late Afternoon on Fatigue in Man: a Preliminary Study." *Neuroscience Letter* 45:317–21. 1984.

Axelrod, J., and Reisine, T. D. "Stress Hormones: Their Interaction and Regulation." *Science* 224:452–59. 1984.

Bartness, T. J., and Goldman, B. D. "Mammalian Pineal Melatonin: A Clock for All Seasons." *Experientia* 45:939–45. 1989.

Bartsch, C., Bartsch, H., Flüchter, S. H., et al. "Diminished Pineal Function Coincides with Disturbed Endocrine Rhythmicity in Untreated Primary Cancer Patients: Consequence of Premature Aging or Tumor Growth?" *Annals of the N.Y. Academy of Science* 719:502–25. 1994.

Bartsch, C., Bartsch, H., Flüchter, S. H., and Lippert, T. H. "Depleted Pineal Melatonin Production in Patients with Primary Breast and Prostate Cancer Is Connected with Circadian Disturbances of Central Hormones: Possible Role of Melatonin for Maintenance and Synchronization of Circadian Rhythmicity." In *Melatonin and the Pineal Gland,* Touitou, Y., Arendt, J., and Pevet, P., eds. 311–16. Elsevier Science Publishers, B.V., 1993.

Bartsch, H., Bartsch, C., Simon, W. E., et al. "Antitumor Activity of the Pineal Gland: Effect of Unidentified Substances Versus the Effect of Melatonin." *Oncology* 49:27–30. 1992.

Beitins, I. Z., Barkan, A., Klibanski, A., et al. "Hormonal Responses to Short Term Fasting in Postmenopausal Women." *Journal of Endocrinology and Metabolism* 60:1120–26. 1985.

Bhattaccharya, S. K., Vivette Glover, I., McIntyre, G., et al. "Stress Causes an Increase in Endogenous Monoamine Oxidase Inhibitor (Tribulin) in Rat Brain." *Neuroscience Letters* 92:218–21. 1988.

Blask, D., and Hill, S. "Effects of Pineal Hormone Melatonin on the Proliferation and Morphological Characteristics of Human Breast Cancer Cells (MCF-7) in Culture." *Cancer Research* 48:6121–26. 1988.

Brugger, P., Marktl, W., and Herold, M. "Impaired Nocturnal Secretion of Melatonin in Coronary Heart Disease." *The Lancet* 945:1408. 1995.

Cohen, M., Lippman, M., and Chabner, B. "Role of Pineal Gland in Etiology and Treatment of Breast Cancer." *The Lancet* 814–16. October 14, 1978.

Covelli, V., Massari, F., and Fallacara, C. "Interleukin-1B and B-Endorphin Circadian Rhythms Are Inversely Related in Normal and Stress-Altered Sleep. *International Journal of Neuroscience* 63:299–305. 1992.

Dahlitz, M. B., Alvarez, J., Vignau, J., English, J., et al. "Delayed Sleep Syndrome Response to Melatonin." *The Lancet* 337:1121–24. 1991.

Danforth, S., Tamarkin, L., and Lippman, M. "Melatonin Increases Oestrogen Receptor Binding Activity of Human Breast Cancer Cells." *Nature* 305: 323–24. 1983.

Selected Bibliography

Dawson, D., and Encel, N. "Melatonin and Sleep in Humans." *Journal of Pineal Research* 15:1–12. 1993.

DeFronzo, R., and Roth, W. "Evidence for the Existence of a Pineal-Adrenal and a Pineal-Thyroid Axis." *Acta Endocrinologica* 70:31–42. 1972.

Demisch, L., Demisch, K., and Nickelsen, T. "Influence of Dexamethasone on Nocturnal Melatonin Production in Healthy Adult Subjects." *Journal of Pineal Research* 5:317–322. 1988.

Dillman, V. M., Anisimov, V. N., Ostroumova, M., et al. "Increase in the Lifespan of Rats Following Polypeptide Pineal Extract Treatment." *Experimental Pathology* 17:539–45. 1979.

Dollins, A., Zhdanova, I., and Wurtman, R. "Effect of Inducing Nocturnal Serum Melatonin Concentrations on Sleep, Mood, Body Temperature and Performance." *Proc. Natl. Acad. Sci, USA.* 91:1824–28. 1994.

Ebling, F. J. B., and Foster, D. L. "Pineal Melatonin Rhythms and Timing of Puberty in Mammals." *Experientia* 45:946–54. 1989.

Ehrlich, S., and Apuzzo, M. L. J. "The Pineal Gland: Anatomy, Physiology, and Clinical Significance." *Journal of Neurosurgery* 63:321–41. 1985.

Esposti, D., Lissoni, P., Tancini, G., et al. "A Study on the Relationship Between the Pineal Gland and the Opiate System in Patients with Cancer." *Cancer* 62:494–99. 1988.

Fabris, N. "Neuroendocrine-Immune Aging: An Integrative View on the Role of Zinc." *Ann. of the N.Y. Acad. of Sci.* 719:353–63. 1994.

———. "A Neuroendocrine-Immune Theory of Aging." *International Journal of Neuroscience* 51:373–75. 1990.

Fabris, N., Amadio, L., Licastro, F., Mocchegiani, E., et al. "Thymic Hormone Deficiency in Normal Aging and Down's Syndrome: Is There a Primary Failure of the Thymus?" *The Lancet* 1:983–86. 1984.

Fabris, N., Mocchegiani, E., Muzzioli, M., and Provincialli, M. "The Role of Zinc in Neuroendocrine-immune Interaction During Aging." *Ann. N.Y. Acad. Sci.* 621:314–26. 1991.

Fabris, N., Pierpaoli, W., and Sorkin, E. "Hormones and the Immunological Capacity. III. The Immunodeficiency Disease of the Hypopituitary Snell-Bagg Dwarf Mice." *Clinical Experimental Immunology* 9:209–25. 1971.

Haimov, I., Laudon, M., and Zisapel, N. "Sleep Disorders and Melatonin Rhythms in Elderly People." *British Medical Journal* 306 (6948): 167ff. 1994.

Hardeland, R., Reiter, R. J., Poeggler, B., and Tan, D. X. "The Significance of the Metabolism of the Neurohormone Melatonin: Antioxidative Protection and Formation of Bioactive Substances." *Neuroscience and Behavioral Reviews* 17:347–57. 1993.

Hastings, M. H., Vance, G., and Maywood, E. "Phylogeny and Function of the Pineal." *Experientia* 45(10):903–1008. 1989.

Heuther, G. "Melatonin Synthesis in the Gastrointestinal Tract and the Impact of Nutritional Factors on Circulating Melatonin." *Ann. of the N.Y. Acad. of Sci.* 719:146–58.

Holloway, W. R., Grota, L. J., and Brown, G. M. "Immunohistochemical Assessment of Melatonin Binding in the Pineal Gland." *Journal of Pineal Research* 2:235–51. 1985.

Irwin, M., Mascovich, A., Gillin, J. C., et al. "Partial Sleep Deprivation Reduces Natural Killer Cell Activity in Humans." *Psychosomatic Medicine* 56(6):493–98. 1994.

Khoory, R., and Stemme, D. "Plasma Melatonin Levels in Patients Suffering from Colorectal Carcinoma." *Journal of Pineal Research* 5:251–58. 1988.

Selected Bibliography

Kobayashi, A. K., Kirschvink, J. L., and Nesson, M. H. "Ferromagnetism and EMFs" (letter) *Nature* 65(18):123. 1995.

Lesnikov, V. A., Isaeva, E. N., Korneva, E., and Pierpaoli, W. "Melatonin Reconstitutes the Decreased CFU-S Content in the Bone Marrow of the Hypothalamus-Lesioned mice." In *Role of Melatonin and Pineal Peptides in Neuroimmunomodulation.* Fraschini, F., and Reiter, R., eds. 225–31. New York: Plenum Press, 1992.

Lesnikov, V. A., Korneva, E. A., Dall'Ara, A., and Pierpaoli, W. "The Involvement of Pineal Gland and Melatonin in Aging. II. Thyrotropin-releasing Hormone and Melatonin Forestall Involution and Promote Reconstitution of the Thymus and Anterior Hypothalamic Area (AHA)-Lesioned mice." *International Journal of Neuroscience* 62:141–53. 1992.

Lesnikov, V. A., and Pierpaoli, W. "Pineal Cross-Transplantation (Old-to-Young and Vice Versa) as Evidence for an Endogenous 'Aging Clock.' " *Ann. of the N.Y. Acad. of Sci.* 719:456–60. 1994.

Lewy, A. J., Wehr, T. A., Goodwin, F. K., et al. "Light Suppresses Melatonin Secretion in Humans." *Science* 210:1267–69.

Lino, A., Silvy, S., Condorelli, L., and Rusconi, A. C. "Melatonin and Jet Lag: Treatment Schedule." *Biol. Psychiatry* 34:587–88. 1993.

Lissoni, P., Barni, S., Cattaneo, E., et al. "Pineal-Interleukin-2 Interactions and Their Possible Importance in the Pathogenesis of Immune Dysfunction in Cancer." In *Role of Melatonin and Pineal Peptides in Neuroimmunomodulation.* Fraschini, E., and Reiter, R., eds. New York: Plenum Press, 1991.

Lissoni, P., Barni, S., Cazzaniga, M., et al. "Efficacy of the Concomitant Administration of the Pineal Hormone Melatonin in Cancer Immunotherapy with Low-Dose IL-2 in Patients with Advanced Solid Tumors

Who Had Progressed on IL-2 Alone." *Oncology* 51:344–47. 1994.

Lissoni, P., Barni, S., Tancini, G., et al. "A Study of the Mechanisms Involved in the Immunostimulatory Action of the Pineal Hormone in Cancer Patients." *Oncology* 50:399–402. 1993.

Lissoni, P., Tancini, G., Barni, S., et al. "Melatonin Increase as Predictor for Tumor Objective Response to Chemotherapy in Advanced Cancer Patients." *Tumori* 4:339–45. 1988.

Loscher, W., Wahnschaffe, U., Lerchl, A., and Stamm, A. "Effects of Weak Alternating Magnetic Fields on Nocturnal Melatonin Production and Mammary Carcinogenesis in Rats." *Oncology* 51:288–95. 1994.

Maestroni, G. J. M., Conti, A., and Pierpaoli, W. "Melatonin, Stress, and the Immune System." *Pineal Research Reviews* 7:203–26. 1989.

———. "Role of Pineal Gland in Immunity III: Melatonin Antagonizes the Immunosuppressive Effect of Acute Stress via an Opiatergic Mechanism." *Immunology* 63:199–204. 1988.

———. "Role of the Pineal Gland in Immunity: Circadian Synthesis and Release of Melatonin Modulates the Antibody Response and Antagonizes the Immunosuppressive Effect of Corticosterone." *Journal of Neuroimmunology* 13:19–30. 1986.

Maestroni, G. J. M., and Pierpaoli, W. "Pharmacologic Control of the Hormonally Mediated Immune Response." In *Psychoneuroimmunology*. New York: Academic Press, 1981.

Masson-Pevet, M., Pevet, P., and Vivien-Roels, B. "Pinealectomy and Constant Release of Melatonin or 5-Methoxtryptamine Induce Testicular Atrophy in the European Hamster. *Journal of Pineal Research* 4:79–88. 1987.

Maurizi, C. P. "Why Not Treat Melancholia with Melatonin and Tryptophan and Treat Seasonal Affective

Selected Bibliography

Disorders with Bright Light?" *Medical Hypotheses* 27:271–76. 1988.

Meyer, B. J., and Theron, J. J. "The Pineal Organ in Man: An Endocrine Gland Awaiting Recognition." *SAMJ.* 73:300–302. 1988.

Miles, A. "Melatonin: Perspectives in the Life Sciences." *Life Sciences* 44:375–85. 1989.

Mocchegiani, E., Bulian, D., Santarelli, L., Tibaldi, A., Muzzioli, M., Pierpaoli, W., and Fabris, N. "The Immuno-Reconstituting Effect of Melatonin or Pineal Grafting and Its Relation to Zinc Pool in Aging Mice." *Journal of Neuroimmunology* 53:189–201. 1994.

Mocchegiani, E., Bulian D., Santarelli, L., Tibaldi, A., Pierpaoli, W., and Fabris, N. "The Zinc-Melatonin Interrelationship: A Working Hypothesis." *Ann. of the N.Y. Acad. of Sci.* 719:298–307.

Morgan, P. J., and Williams, L. M. "Central Melatonin Receptors: Implications for a Mode of Action." *Experientia* 45:955–64. 1989.

Nakazawa, K., Marubayashi, U., and McCann, S. M. "Mediation of the Short-Loop Negative Feedback of Luteinizing Hormone (LH) on LH-Releasing Hormone Release by Melatonin-Induced Inhibition of LH Release from the Pars Tuberalis." *Proc. Natl. Acad. Sci. USA* 88:7576–79. 1991.

Natsuko, M., Aoyama, H., Murase, T., and Mori, W. "Anti-Hypercholesterolemic Effect of Melatonin in Rats." *Acta Pathologica Japonica* 39(10): 613–18.

"NIA Consensus Development Conference: The Treatment of Sleep Disorders in Older People." *NIA Research Bulletin* (September 1990).

"NIA Funds Timely Research on Sleep, Melatonin and the Circadian Clock." *NIA Research Bulletin* (July 1992).

Penny, R. "Episodic Secretion of Melatonin in Pre- and Postpubertal Girls and Boys." *Journal of Clinical Endocrinology and Metabolism* 60:751–56. 1985.

Selected Bibliography

Penny, R., Stanczyk, F., and Goebelsmann, U. "Melatonin: Data Consistent with a Role in Controlling Ovarian Function." *J. Endocrinol. Invest.* 10:499–505. 1987.

Pierpaoli, W. "Changes of the Hormonal Status in Young Mice by Restricted Caloric Diet: Relation to Lifespan Extension." Preliminary Results. *Experientia* 33:1612–13. 1977.

———. "Inability of Thymus Cells from Newborn Donors to Restore Transplantation Immunity in Athymic Mice." *Immunology* 29:323–38. 1975.

———. "Integrated Phylogenetic and Ontogenetic Evolution of Neuroendocrine and Identity-Defence, Immune Functions." In *Psychoneuroimmunology.* Ader, R., ed. 575–606. New York: Academic Press, 1981.

———. "The Pineal Aging Clock: Evidence, Models, and an Approach to Age-Delaying Strategies." In *Aging, Immunity and Infection.* Powers, D. C., Morley, J. E., and Coe, R. M., eds. New York: Springer Publishing, 1993.

———. "The Pineal Gland: A Circadian or a Seasonal Aging Clock?" *Aging* 3:99–101. 1991.

———. "Pineal Grafting and Melatonin Induce Immunocompetence in Nude (Athymic) Mice." *Int. J. Neurosci.* 68:123–31. 1993.

Pierpaoli, W., and Besedovsky, H. O. "Failure of the 'Thymus Factor' to Restore Transplantation Immunity in Athymic Mice." *Brit. J. Exp. Path.* 56:180–82. 1975.

———. "Role of the Thymus in Programming of Neuroendocrine Functions." *Clin. Exp. Immunol.* 20:328–38. 1975.

Pierpaoli, W., Bianchi, E., and Sorkin, E. "Hormones and the Immunological Capacity. V. Modification of Growth Hormone Producing Cells in the Adenohophysis of Neonatally Thymectomized Germ-Free Mice: An Electron Microscope Study." *Clin. Exp. Immunol.* 9:889–901. 1971.

Selected Bibliography

Pierpaoli, W., Dall'Ara, A., Pedrinis E., and Regelson, W. "The Pineal Control of Aging: The Effects of Melatonin and Pineal Grafting on the Survival of Older Mice." *Ann. N.Y. Acad. of Sci.* 621:291–313. 1991.*

Pierpaoli, W., Fabris, N., and Sorkin, E. "Developmental Hormones and Immunological Maturation. In *Hormones and the Immune Response*. Ciba Foundation Study Group No. 36. Cohen, S., Cudkowicz, G., McCluskey, R. T., eds. Basel: Karger, 1971.

Pierpaoli, W., Haemmerli, M., Sorkin, E., and Hurni, H. "Role of the Thymus and Hypothalamus in Aging." In *V. European Symposium on Basic Research in Gerontology*. Schmidt, U. J., Bruschke, G., Lang E., et al., eds. 141–50. Erlangen, Germany: Verlag Dr. Med. Straube, 1976.

Pierpaoli, W., Kopp, H. G., Muller, J., and Keller, M. "Interdependence Between Neuroendocrine Programming and the Generation of Immune Recognition in Ontogeny." *Cell Immun*. 29:16–27. 1977.

Pierpaoli, W., and Maestroni, G. "Melatonin: A Principal Neuroimmunoregulatory and Anti-Stress Hormone. Its Anti-Aging Effects." *Immunol. Lett*. 16:-355–62. 1987.

* In this article, we make reference to an isolated experiment in which the test mice later developed ovarian cancer and cancers of the reproductive tract. Subsequent research in the field has allayed any earlier concerns we might have had about the use of melatonin by younger women. We now believe that the particular breed of mice was prone to cancers of this type and that the melatonin treatments were only coincidental. The evidence is overwhelming that melatonin, even at very high dosages, is safe. In particular, we refer you to work of Dr. Michael Cohen of Applied Medical Research Ltd., which is discussed in detail in Chapter 10. To obtain FDA approval, Dr. Cohen has done extensive rigorous testing of melatonin in animals and humans. In Holland, over 2,000 women have been taking 75 mg of melatonin daily for more than three years. The results of these studies on animals and humans has demonstrated that melatonin is not only safe, but actually has a protective effect against some cancers. Based on evidence not available to us at the time of writing this paper, we have absolutely no reservations about recommending melatonin to adults.

Selected Bibliography

Pierpaoli, W., and Meshorer, A. "Host Endocrine Status Mediates Oncogenesis: Leukemia Virus-Induced Carcinomas and Reticulum Cell Sarcomas in Acyclic or Normal Mice." *Eur. J. Cancer Clin. Oncol.* 18(11): 1181–85. 1982.

Pierpaoli, W., and Regelson, W. "Pineal Control of Aging: Effect of Melatonin and Pineal Grafting on Aging Mice." *Proc. Natl. Acad. of Sci. USA* 94:787–91. 1994.

Pierpaoli W., and Sorkin, E. "Alternations of Adrenal Cortex and Thyroid in Mice with Congenital Absence of the Thymus." *Nature New Biology* 238:282–85. 1972.

———. "Cellular Modifications in the Hypophysis of Neonatally Thymectomized Mice." *Brit. J. Exp. Path.* 49:288–93. 1968.

———. "Effect of Gonadectomy on the Peripheral Lymphatic Tissue of Neonatally Thymectomized Mice." *Brit. J. Exp. Path.* 49:288–93. 1968.

———. "Effect of Growth Hormone and Anti-Growth Hormone Serum on the Lymphatic Tissue and the Immune Response." *Antibiotica et Chemotherapia* 15:122–34. Sorkin, E., ed. Basel: Karger-Verlag, 1969.

———. "Hormones, Thymus and Lymphocyte Functions." *Experientia* 28:1385–89. 1972.

———. "Relationship Between Thymus and Hypophysis." *Nature* 215:834–37. 1967.

———. "A Study on Anti-Pituitary Serum." *Immunology* 16:311–18. 1969.

Pierpaoli, W., and Yi, C. X. "The Involvement of Pineal Gland and Melatonin in Immunity and Aging. I. Thymus-Mediated, Immunoreconstituting and Antiviral Activity of Thyrotropin-releasing Hormone." *J. Neuroimmunolo.* 27:99–109. 1990.

———. "The Pineal Gland and Melatonin: The Aging Clock? A Concept and Experimental Evidence." In *Stress and the Aging Brain: Integrative Mechanisms.*

Selected Bibliography

Nappi, G., Genazzani, A. R., Martignoni, E., and Petraglia, F., eds. 172–75, New York: Raven Press, 1990.

Prechel, M. M., Audhya T. K., Swenson R., et. al. "A Seasonal Pineal Peptide Rhythm Persists in Superior Cervical Ganglionectomized Rats." *Life Sciences* 44:103–10. 1989.

Rahamimoff, R., and Bruderman, I. "Changes in Pulmonary Mechanics Induced by Melatonin." *Life Sciences* 4:1383–89. 1965.

Regelson, W., and Kalimi, M. "Dehydroepiandrosterone (DHEA)—The Multifunctional Steroid. II. Effects on CNS, Cell Proliferation, Metabolic and Vascular, Clinical and Other Effects. Mechanism of Action?" *Ann. of the N.Y. Acad. of Sci.* 719:564–75. 1994.

Regelson, W., and Pierpaoli, W. "Melatonin: A Rediscovered Antitumor Hormone? Its Relation to Surface Receptors; Sex Steroid Metabolism, Immunologic Response, and Chronobiologic Factors in Tumor Growth and Therapy." *Cancer Investigation* 5(4):379–85. 1987.

Regelson, W. and Sinex, F. N., eds. *Intervention and the Aging Process; Part A: Quantitation Epidemiology and Clinical Research; Part B: Basic Research and Pre-clinical Screening.* New York: Alan R. Liss, 1983.

Reiter, R. J. "Neuroendocrinology of Melatonin." In *Melatonin, Clinical Perspectives.* Miles, A., Philbrick, D. R. S., and Thompson, C., eds. 1–5. Oxford: Oxford University Press, 1988.

———. "Pineal Melatonin: Cell Biology of Its Synthesis and of Its Physiological Interactions." *Endocrine Reviews* 12:151–80. 1991.

Reiter, R. J., Tan, D. X., Pöeggeler, B., et al. "Melatonin as a Free Radical Scavenger: Implications for Aging and Age-Related Diseases." *Ann. of the N.Y. Acad. of Sci.* 719:1–12. 1994.

Reppert, S. M., Weaver, D., Rivkees, S., and Stopa, E.

Selected Bibliography

"Putative Melatonin Receptors in Human Biological Clock." *Science* 242:78–82. 1988.

Rosenthal, N. E., Sack, D. A., Carpenter, C. J., et al. "Antidepressant Effects of Light in Seasonal Depression." *Am. J. Psychiatry* 142:163–70. 1985.

Rosenthal, N. E., Sack, D. A., and Wehr, T. A. "Seasonal Variations in Affective Disorders." In *Circadian Rhythms in Psychiatry*. Wehr, T. A., and Goodwin, F. K., eds. 185–201. New York: Academic Press, 1983.

Rozencwaig, R., Grad, B. R., and Ochoa, J. "The Role of Melatonin and Serotonin in Aging." *Medical Hypotheses* 23:337–52. 1987.

Samples, J. R., Krause, G., Lewy, A. J., "Effect of Melatonin on Intraocular Pressure." *Current Eye Research* 7(7):649–53. 1988.

Sandyk, R. "Melatonin and the Maturation of REM Sleep." *Intern. J. Neuroscience* 63:105–14.

Schalger, D. "Early-Morning Administration of Short Acting B-Blockers for Treatment of Winter Depression." *Am. J. Psychiatry* 151(9):1383–85. 1994.

Scuderi, P. "Differential Effect of Copper and Zinc on Human Peripheral Blood Monocyte Cytokine Secretion." *Cell Immunol.* 126:391–405. 1990.

Shirama, K., Furuya, T., Takeo, Y., et al. "Direct Effect of Melatonin on the Accessory Sexual Organs in Pinealectomized Male Rats Kept in Constant Darkness." *Journal of Endocrinology* 95:87–94. 1982.

Souêtre, E., Rosenthal, N., and Ortonne J. P. "Affective Disorders, Light and Melatonin." *Photodermatology* 5:107–9. 1988.

Souêtre, E., Salvati, E., Belugou, J. L., et al. "5-Methoxypsoralen Increases Evening Sleepiness in Humans: Possible Involvement of the Melatonin Secretion." *Eur. J. Clin. Pharmacol.* 36:91–92. 1989.

Takahashi, J. S., and Katz, M. "Regulation of Circadian Rhythmicity." *Science* 217:1104–11. 1982.

Tan, D. A., Pöeggeler, B., Reiter, R., et al. "The Pineal

Selected Bibliography

Hormone Melatonin Inhibits DNA-Adduct Formation Induced by the Chemical Carcinogen Safrole In Vivo." *Cancer Lett.* 70:65–71. 1993.

Touitou, Y., Bogdan, A., and Auzéby, A. "Activity of Melatonin and Other Pineal Indoles on the In Vitro Synthesis of Cortisol, Cortisone, and Adrenal Androgens." *Journal of Pineal Research* 6:341–50. 1989.

Touitou, Y., Fèvre, M., Lagoguey, M., et al. "Age and Mental Health–Related Circadian Rhythms of Plasma Melatonin, Prolactin, Luteinizing Hormone and Follicle-stimulating Hormone in Man." *Journal of Endocrinology* 91:467–75. 1981.

Touitou, Y., Fèvre-Montange, M., Proust, J., et al. "Age- and Sex-Associated Modification of Plasma Melatonin Concentrations in Man. Relationship to Pathology, Malignant or Not, and Autopsy Findings." *Acta Endocrinologica* 108:135–44. 1985.

Touitou, Y., and Haus, E. "Aging of the Human Endocrine and Neuroendocrine Time Structure." *Ann. of the N.Y. Acad. of Sci.* 719:378–97. 1994.

Troiani, M. E., Reiter, R. J., Vaughan, M. K., et al. "Swimming Depresses Nighttime Melatonin Content Without Changing N-Acetyltransferase Activity in the Rat Pineal Gland." *Neuroendocrinology* 47:55–60. 1988.

Underwood, H. "The Pineal and Melatonin: Regulators of Circadian Function in Lower Vertebrates." *Experientia* 45:914–22. 1989.

Voorduow, B., Euser, R., Verdonk, R., et al. "Melatonin and Melatonin-Progestin Combinations Alter Pituitary Ovarian Function in Women and Can Inhibit Ovulation." *Journal of Clinical Endocrinology and Metabolism* 74(1):108–17. 1992.

Waldhauser, F., Ehrhart, B., and Forster, E. "Clinical Aspects of the Melatonin Action: Impact of Development, Aging, and Puberty, Involvement of Melatonin in Psychiatric Disease and Importance of Neuroimmu-

Selected Bibliography

noendocrine Interactions." *Neuroimmunology Review* 671–81. 1993.

Weiss, J. M., Sundar, S. K., Becker, K. J., and Cierpial, M. A. "Behavioral and Neural Influences on Cellular Immune Responses: Effects of Stress and Interleukin-1." *J. Clin. Psychiatry* 50 (No. 5, Suppl.):43–53. 1989.

Wilson, B. "Chronic Exposure to ELF Fields May Induce Depression." *Bioelectromagnetics* 9:195–205. 1988.

Wirz-Justice, A., Graw, P., and Krauchi, K. "Light Therapy in Seasonal Affective Disorder Is Independent of Time of Day or Circadian Phase." *Arch. Gen. Psychiatry* 50:929–37. 1993.

Wurtman, R. J. "Fall in Nocturnal Serum Melatonin Levels During Prepuberty and Prepubescence." *The Lancet* 362–85. 1984.

———"The Pineal as a Neuroendocrine Transducer." *Hospital Practice* (January 1980) 82–91.

Wurtman, R. J., and Lieberman, H. "Melatonin Secretion as a Mediator of Circadian Variations in Sleep and Sleepiness." *Journal of Pineal Research* 2:301–3. 1985.

Wurtman, R. J., and Wurtman, J. J. "Carbohydrates and Depression." *Scientific American* 260(1):68–74. 1989.

Wutian, W., Chen, Y., and Reiter, R. J. "Day-Night Differences in the Response of the Pineal Gland to Swimming Stress." *Proceedings of the Society for Experimental Biology and Medicine* 187:315–19. 1988.

Young, I., Francis, P., Leone, A., et al. "Constant Pineal Output and Increasing Mass Account for Declining Melatonin Levels During Human Growth and Sexual Maturation." *Journal of Pineal Research* 5:71–85. 1988.

Zisapel, N. "Melatonin Receptors Revisited." *Journal of Neural Transmission* 73:1–5. 1988.

INDEX

acquired immune deficiency
    syndrome (AIDS), 102,
    104, 155–60
    illnesses related to, 102,
        115, 123, 156, 157
    melatonin and, 100, 119,
        155, 157, 158–60
    prevention of, 157
    risk factors for, 105, 156
    T cells and, 30, 105, 157–
        58, 159, 160
    tests for, 156
    transmission of, 156–57
    see also human
        immunodeficiency virus
adenosine triphosphate
    (ATP), 92–93, 152–53
adrenal glands, 27–28, 35, 36,
    87, 114, 151, 159, 198,
    199, 200
    adrenaline, 27–28, 114,
        151
aging clock, xvi, xix, 6–7, 19,
    253
    breakdown of, 8–9, 10–11
    discovery of, 3–7, 10–11,
        18, 20–21, 29, 37, 43, 62,
        181, 255
    resetting of, 6, 10, 82, 83–
        96, 101

search for, 29–48
    see also pineal gland
Aging Clock, The, 90
aging process:
    acceleration of, 30, 32, 41,
        47–48, 49
    control of, xxi, 6–7, 9, 26,
        30, 32, 35, 50, 53
    delay of, xv, xvi, xx, xxi,
        4, 6–7, 8–11, 49–54
    hormones and, 27, 86–87
    illness associated with, xvi,
        5–6, 8–9, 16–17, 50, 85,
        87, 94, 117, 160–64, 169,
        237, 254–56
    loss of identity and, 104
    melatonin and, xvi, xix–
        xxi, 6–7, 8, 10–15, 16,
        40–41, 47–62, 69, 73–
        75, 83–96, 117, 206,
        235–40
    outward vs. inward
        manifestation of, 13, 78–
        79, 103
    physical deterioration and,
        xviii, 4–6, 8–9, 10–11,
        13–14, 18, 20, 41, 61, 79,
        83, 117, 254
    research on, xvi–xxi, 4,
        6–7, 16–17, 22

Index

Index

breast cancer (*cont.*)
  risk factors for, 127, 137–
    40, 141, 191, 194
  treatment of, 14, 120, 125,
    127–30
breast feeding, 8, 73, 156, 236
  letdown response and, 82
breast milk, 8, 73, 184, 185
bronchodilators, 165
"bubble" children, 34
Burnet, F. M., 106

caesarean section, 34
calcitonin, 77
calcium, 77, 79, 93, 126, 152–
  53
cancer, 23, 94, 100, 104
  cholesterol and, 146
  deaths from, 11, 122
  diet and, 15, 108, 135
  electromagnetic fields and,
    67
  hormone-dependent, 124–
    30
  immune system breakdown
    and, 121–25
  increasing rates of, xviii,
    122, 135
  melatonin and, xix, xxi,
    14–15, 16, 50, 69, 85, 96,
    99, 118–19, 120–42, 242,
    248
  metastasis of, 124, 125,
    128
  obesity and, 127, 250–51
  prevention of, xviii, xix,
    xxi, 85, 96, 99, 118–19,
    120–21, 122, 140–42, 242
  quality of life and, 121,
    132–33

research on, xvii–xviii, 10–
    11, 14–15, 24–25, 120,
    121, 126–28
  resistance to, 100, 104, 106,
    120–42
  risk factors for, 25, 67, 87,
    89, 93–94, 101, 108, 121,
    122, 124–25, 126, 135–40,
    196, 247
  treatment of, xviii, 14, 128–
    35
  see also tumors; *specific
    cancers*
Candida albicans, 105
carbohydrates, 166–67, 229,
  234
carcinogens, 90, 95, 124, 128,
  135, 242, 248
carotenes, 90, 120
Case, J. D., 68, 216
cataracts, 49, 89, 173–74
cells:
  division of, 89, 124, 129
  foreign, 46, 102, 106, 107, 111
  membranes of, 89, 90, 124
  memory, 103, 107, 109–10,
    111, 131
  mutation of, 124
  oxidative damage to, 88,
    89–90, 91, 92
cerebral cortex, 58*n*, 199
chameleons, 69
chemotherapy, xviii, 14, 128–
    34
  melatonin combined with,
    129–35, 141
  nighttime intravenous
    delivery of, 134
  side effects of, 129, 131–32,
    133–34

Index

Index

Index

Index

revival of, 7, 10, 33, 36, 38, 82, 83, 101, 103–04, 113, 116, 118
sex and, 35–37, 39, 45
stress and, 25, 76, 114, 143, 197–200, 202–07
thymus gland and, 33–37, 56, 109, 115
thyroid gland and, 35, 108
see also acquired immune deficiency syndrome; autoimmune diseases
immunization, 17, 23, 106, 111, 112, 197
immunoglobulins, 106
immunology, xvii, 3, 6, 22–24, 25, 40
immunosurveillance, 106, 109
immunotherapy, xviii, 14
impotency, 190
infection, 159
resistance to, 30, 95, 100, 103, 106, 107, 110–13
see also bacteria; viruses
influenza, 25
insomnia, 14, 164, 193, 207, 208, 217, 218, 219, 221, 238, 241, 243, 244
insulin, 166–68, 242
insulin resistance, 167–68
interleukin-2 (IL-2), 131–32
iodine, 187
Irwin, Michael, 210

Jankovic, Branislav D., 29, 58n
jet lag, 14, 65, 223–27, 234, 238, 245–46
Journal of Reproductive Rhythms, The, 71

Kaposi's sarcoma, 123
kidneys, 27, 35, 55, 75, 86, 114, 149, 199
cancer of, 131, 132–48
function of, 150
transplanting of, 24

Lancet, 126
laser surgery, 175
Lerner, A. B., 68, 216
Lesnikov, Vladimir, 58–61, 134
leukemia, 135
life span:
extension of, 3–5, 7, 9, 11, 17, 18, 40, 48–50, 52–62, 100, 110, 118, 197, 250
light and, 40–41
of men vs. women, 67
quality of life and, 53, 118
shortening of, 30, 33, 38, 41, 48, 242
lifestyle, 122, 135, 141, 206, 246
light:
artificial, 41, 47, 65, 72, 135–36
cycles of dark and, 7–8, 39–41, 64–67, 211–16, 218, 223–24
disorders related to, 223–34
melatonin and, 47–48, 64–65, 69–70, 72, 135–36, 211–12, 230–34
pineal gland and, 7, 8, 40–41, 47–48, 63–69, 80, 211–12, 223
therapeutic role of, 231–34
ultraviolet, 90, 124
Lissoni, Paoli, 131–32

307

Index

liver, 91, 95, 132, 145, 242
Longevity, 196
low-density lipoprotein
    (LDL), 146–47
lung cancer, 122
lungs, 107, 164–65
luteinizing hormone (LH), 74,
    184
lymphatic system, 124
lymphocytes, 24, 36, 104,
    105, 112, 203
    see also B lymphocytes;
    T lymphocytes
lymphomas, 123

macrophages, 107
macular degeneration, 175–77
manic disorder, 231
Marshall, Barry, xix
maternal instinct, 64–65, 73,
    82, 184, 185, 194
measles, 106
meat, 146, 252
melanoma, 132
melatonin:
    animal-based, 17
    antioxidant capacity of, 88–
      91, 153–54, 173
    availability and cost of, xvi,
      6, 17–18, 239, 252
    biological production of,
      xvi, 7, 8, 16, 40, 41, 47,
      53, 63–71, 80, 94, 135,
      183
    brands of, 20
    declining levels of, 8–9, 12,
      47–48, 53, 69, 74, 80, 84–
      87, 93, 118, 121, 126–27,
      168, 237
    discovery of, 68–69, 216

    dosages of, 12, 86, 118, 142,
      160, 171, 191, 192–93, 216,
      219–20, 237–40, 243–46
    function of, xvi, 8, 70–71,
      75–77, 84, 86–88, 168
    gender differences and, 72
    hormones regulated by, 86–
      87, 91, 168, 191–92
    nighttime secretion of, 7,
      47, 53, 64, 67, 69, 73,
      117, 126, 134, 135, 208,
      211, 223, 231, 248
    non-prescription status of,
      xvi, 17–18
    research on, xxi, 10–18, 41,
      46–62, 68–69, 82, 84
    safety of, xxi, 6, 17, 209
    slow-release form of, 218
    as state-dependent
      hormone, 75
    sublingual form of, 240
    supplements of, xvi, 6, 12,
      48–54, 62, 69, 84–87, 95,
      99, 101, 115, 118, 121,
      147–48, 164, 184, 188–89,
      208, 235–52
    synthetic form of, xvi, 18,
      240
"Melatonin As a Free Radical
    Scavenger" (Reiter), 90–
    91
memory, xxi, 151, 162, 251
    cell, 103, 107, 109–10, 111,
      130
    loss of, 161, 162, 164, 171,
      203
menopause, 27, 52, 75, 81,
    186, 208
    HRT for, 12, 161, 193–94,
      244

Index

Index

quality of life, 3–4, 9, 53, 117–18, 121, 132

rapid eye movement (REM), 14, 170, 183, 212–14, 217
Regelson, William, xv*n*, xxii, 15, 21–24, 55, 90, 121
Reiter, Russell, 90–91, 130, 139, 242
renal cancer, 131, 133
renal cell carcinoma, 133
renin, 150
reproduction, 37, 42, 45, 82, 86
 animal, 7–10, 41, 45, 46–47, 70–71, 73, 81
 death and, 9–10
 delay of, 169, 186
 genetic transmission and, 45
 human fertility peaks and, 71–72
 melatonin and, 70–72, 75, 186–88
 see also sexuality
reptiles, 66, 69
retina, 63, 80, 173, 211
 detached, 175
retrolental fibrosis, 40
retroviruses, 156
rheumatoid arthritis, 101, 108, 196
Rosenthal, Norman E., 228, 232
Ross, Steven, 128
Rudenstine, Neil, 195

sanitation, 197
sarcomas, 121–22, 123
Savalas, Telly, 128

seasonal affective disorder (SAD), 224, 227–34
seasons, 7–8, 39–40, 64–65
 animal breeding and, 70–71
 human fertility and, 71–72
 weather changes and, 7–8, 39, 64–65, 66, 70–71, 72, 77–78
 see also seasonal affective disorder
selenium, 89
Selye, Hans, 197–99, 201
semen, 156, 189
Semmelweis, Ignaz Philipp, xix
senescence, 5, 38, 49, 50, 80, 156, 256
serotonin, 80–81, 229
serotonin uptake inhibitors, 80
sexuality:
 development of, 20, 26, 31, 35, 44, 63, 68, 69, 186, 251
 diminished function and, 75, 181–82, 184, 186, 188–90, 205
 hormones and, 10, 20, 26, 28, 31, 35–37, 52, 75, 145, 182–86, 191–92
 immune system and, 35–37, 39, 45
 libido and, 45, 183–85, 187, 194, 229
 melatonin and, xxi, 7, 11, 52, 69, 70–72, 74–75, 181–94
 rejuvenation of, xxi, 7, 11, 52, 116, 182–83, 186
 synchronicity and, 190–91

311

Index

Index

Index